CAESAREAN BIRTH IN BRITAIN

Caesarean Birth in Britain

Dr Colin Francome, Professor Wendy Savage,
Helen Churchill, Helen Lewison

MIDDLESEX UNIVERSITY PRESS
Published in association with
The National Childbirth Trust

© Dr Colin Francome, Professor Wendy Savage, Helen Churchill,
Helen Lewison and the National Childbirth Trust 1993

First published in 1993 by Middlesex University Press.
Middlesex University Press is an imprint of Middlesex University Services Limited,
Bounds Green Road, London N11 2NQ.

A CIP Catalogue record for this book is available
from the British Library

ISBN 1 898253 00 5

Illustrations, with the exception of those on
pages 11 and 16, by Helen Chown

Editorial, design and production in association with
Book Production Consultants, 25–27 High Street,
Chesterton, Cambridge CB4 1ND
Typeset in Sabon by Rowland Phototypesetting Limited,
Bury St Edmunds, Suffolk and printed by
The Alden Press, Osney Mead, Oxford.

CONTENTS

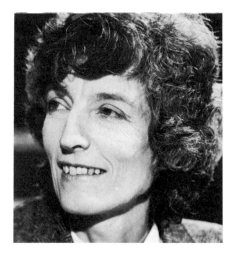

PROFESSOR WENDY SAVAGE is Consultant Obstetrician at the Royal London Hospital and Visiting Professor in Health at Middlesex University. She has written numerous articles for the major medical journals and published books for both academics and the general public. She is widely regarded as one of the leading advocates of women's rights in Britain.

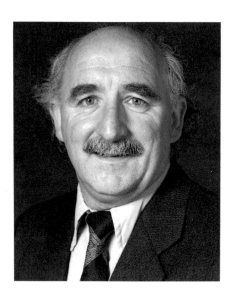

DR COLIN FRANCOME became interested in the increasing caesarean section rate in 1978 when his daughter was born in a hospital in New York where one in four births was by this method. He has published books on a wide variety of subjects, including the environment, juggling, clowning, abortion and caesarean rates. He has had articles published in many of the major British journals including *BMJ*, *Lancet*, *British Journal of Criminology* and *Political Quarterly*. Dr Francome is a reader at Middlesex University.

HELEN LEWISON was a solicitor before the birth of her two children, now aged eleven and eight. She has worked as a volunteer for the NCT in many capacities for more than ten years, and is currently Chairman of the Council of Trustees and an antenatal teacher. She wrote *Your Choices for Pregnancy and Childbirth* for the NCT in association with *Good Housekeeping* magazine and was one of the contributors to *The NCT Book of Pregnancy, Birth and Parenthood*, edited by Glynnis Tucker. She has served as a member of her local Maternity Services Liaison Committee for four years and has a particular interest in working to make maternity services more appropriate to women's needs.

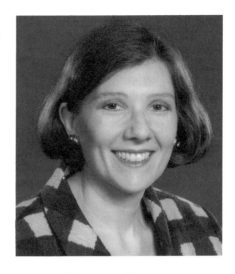

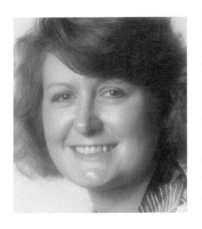

HELEN CHURCHILL is a senior lecturer and health studies subject leader at the Crewe + Alsager Faculty of the Manchester Metropolitan University. She is the only one of the authors to have had a baby by caesarean and has delved deeply into both the history of the operation and the experiences of women giving birth by this method. She has nearly completed a PhD in this area at Middlesex University.

ACKNOWLEDGEMENTS

Helen Lewison would like to acknowledge the comments and support of Bridget Baker, Patricia Donnithorne, Christine Glossop, Alex Hunter and Carole Warren and also the practical support of her husband Kim Lewison.

Helen Churchill would like to thank Leah, Barbara and the rest of her family for their support. She would also like to thank all the women who participated in the study, gave their time and took the trouble to answer the questions at a time when they were probably not feeling at their best.

Colin Francome would like to thank Cathy Doggrell, Debbie Miller, Pat Garrat, Maureen Burton, Maggie Padden-Smith, Carla Francome, William Francome, Viv Williamson, Norma Smailes, Julie Clark, Julie Lau, the Royal College of Midwives, and the Nuffield Foundation for a grant towards some of the research.

Wendy Savage would like to thank Helen Cagnoni, Jay Savage and Bob Davenport for their help in various different ways.

We would all like to thank Suzanne Dobson of the NCT and also Joe Ormerod, for choosing this book to be the first-ever publication of Middlesex University Press; Roz Williams, Debbie Wayment and Stephanie Zarach at Book Production Consultants; and Helen Chown for the illustrations.

CHAPTER ONE

INTRODUCTION

The differences in caesarean rates between countries and regions cannot be explained by the physical characteristics of the women and they therefore raise serious ethical and economic considerations.

WOMEN are almost three times more likely to have a caesarean birth now than they were twenty years ago. In 1973 the estimated caesarean rate for England and Wales was 5.3 per cent and our recent survey shows a probable rate for Britain in 1992 of 13 per cent.

We have written this book because we are of the opinion that many caesareans are being performed unnecessarily. At the beginning of the twentieth century, some obstetricians were concerned about the then rising rates and brought up the same issues that we deal with in this book. At the end of the twentieth century, rates have risen much higher, but there is little public debate about them and a worrying lack of concern in many quarters. We aim to inform and promote such a debate between all interested parties, but particularly women, who are the ones who have to undergo the operation and its attendant risks and cope with its aftermath, in addition to caring for a new baby. We therefore hope that this book will be read by women and their families as well as health professionals and antenatal teachers.

One factor contributing to the lack of debate may be the paucity of accurate official statistics. The latest official government statistics date from 1985, showing a rate for England and Wales of 10.5 per cent. In reply to a parliamentary question on 1 March 1993 relating to the number of caesarean births, Tom Sackville MP, Parliamentary Secretary for Health, replied that 'there are no data for the years 1986 to 1987–8'. The estimated rate for 1990–91 from the Hospital Episode Statistics was 13 per cent: '(These are broad estimates based on incomplete date, and are rounded to the nearest 1,000)' (Hansard 1.3.1993, col. 29/30). Since each maternity unit collates its own intervention rates for internal audit and for the information of district health authorities purchasing maternity services, it is surprising that these cannot be collected and collated manually until the new coding system for National Health Service (NHS) statistics is in force. The Royal College of Obstetricians and Gynaecologists also collects national figures each year and these could be made available.

There is no doubt that some doctors have seen caesarean sections as the birthing method of the future. In this respect, it is instructive to quote from an article by Sutherst and Case:[1]

> It may well be that during the next forty years the allowing of a vaginal delivery or attempted vaginal delivery may need to be justified in each particular instance. Perhaps it is not altogether too provocative to suggest that vaginal delivery may yet become the exception rather than the rule.

This is not the first time, by any means, that unnecessary surgery has been carried out. We can recall the great increase in tonsillectomies which began in the late 1920s and persisted at a high rate for thirty years until an outbreak of poliomyelitis in the 1950s led to the postponement of many operations and the eventual realisation that for many children the operation was not necessary.

Oakley and Richards make two interesting points of relevance here:[2]

> In the context of medical attitudes towards Caesarean sections, it would seem to be of some significance that they are referred to, and discussed, in a rather different way than other forms of abdominal surgery . . . We do not call it a Caesarean 'operation', Caesarean 'surgery', or even a hysterotomy [cut in the uterus], but we use the rather odd, but perhaps benign, term 'section' . . . Thus, while it is accepted among surgeons that depression is a common consequence of major surgery (especially of emergency surgery), the same assumption is not made about Caesarean section.

The lack of concern among many obstetricians about the after-effects of the rising caesarean rates may result from the fact that they spend little time postnatally with women who have had caesarean sections and are far removed from any physical or psychological ill-effects resulting from the operation. A 1988 study showed that low emotional well-being and negative feelings about the baby were both associated with having had a caesarean.[3] More women were likely to describe their caesarean birth as 'fulfilling' if it was performed under epidural anaesthesia. This was also the finding in our own survey of women's experiences (see Chapter 7) and yet it can be seen

....

1 Sutherst and Case, 1975, p. 259.
2 Oakley and Richards, 1990, p. 191.
3 Green, Coupland and Kitzinger, 1988.

from our survey of consultants (see Chapter 8) that epidural anaesthesia is often not available even for elective caesareans.

In another study women were interviewed six months after delivery, and it was found that women delivered by emergency caesarean section took significantly longer than those who gave birth vaginally to feel close to their babies.[4] A further study of women who gave birth by caesarean found that only 87 per cent of women were able to give the correct reasons for their operation.[5] At three months after the operation, 35 per cent felt they had still not fully recovered; 28 per cent felt less healthy than before the pregnancy; and 38 per cent had depression. There also appears to be a failure to appreciate the deep and lasting nature of women's memories and feelings about their births which can continue for many years.[6]

REASONS FOR THE RISE AND VARIATION IN RATES OF CAESAREAN SECTION

There are some perfectly good reasons for the rise in caesarean rates. The operation is much safer than it was and one important factor for the increase, consultants told us, is the improvements in anaesthetic techniques. However, there are wide differences in practice between different countries. Women in the United States are almost twice as likely to have a caesarean as women in Britain. Nearly a quarter of American deliveries are now performed by caesarean.[7] From our latest data it is believed that the rate in the United States has reached a plateau, but in England and Wales it appears still to be rising.

The differences in caesarean rates between countries and regions cannot be explained by the physical characteristics of the women and they therefore raise serious ethical and economic considerations. If the high level of caesareans in the United States were due to better medical practice, more accurate diagnosis and better management of labour problems, leading to healthier mothers and babies, then there would be a strong case for an increase in the caesarean rate in Britain. However, we know that both the maternal and perinatal mortality rates in the United States are higher than in Britain, despite the fact that the United States is materially more wealthy.

If, as this suggests, the US rate is high because of non-medical reasons such as doctors being frightened of being sued for negligence, it would

....

4 Hillan, 1992a.
5 Hillan, 1992b.
6 Simkin, 1991.
7 Taffel, Placek and Kosary, 1992.

suggest that women in the United States are undergoing a great deal of unnecessary surgery. In fact, one estimate is that each year over 144 women die in the United States from unnecessary operations.[8]

BRITISH OBSTETRIC CARE   In Britain, unlike in North America, most deliveries are carried out by midwives who are trained as sole practitioners in their own right. Women in Britain have the right to have a baby at home and about 1 per cent of births are home deliveries. However, the overall responsibility for the vast majority of births is perceived to lie with approximately 800 consultant obstetricians. These consultants head teams, formerly known as 'firms'. These are hierarchical groups which usually include doctors at various stages of training and experience known as senior registrars, registrars and senior house officers (SHOs). (Some hospital protocols use the phrase 'chain of command' in describing situations when appropriate medical assistance should be sought.) The SHO will be someone at the first level of their formal training who may rarely do some normal deliveries in conjunction with the midwives. The higher-level doctors will be called in if there are any problems and will perform caesareans. In a typical British maternity unit there will be any number of consultants from two to ten and they will meet periodically to discuss such issues as perinatal deaths. General practitioners (GPs) can also carry out deliveries either in conjunction with a consultant unit or independently, either at home or in a GP- or midwife-led unit. However, if a caesarean should become necessary, this will almost always be carried out under a consultant's authority and women may have to be transferred to a larger unit from a small unit or from home should the need for a caesarean arise.

VARIATIONS IN CAESAREAN RATES IN BRITAIN   Reports within the countries in Britain also show considerable variation in rates. In 1989 there was a rate of 12.1 per cent in England, 13.5 per cent in Wales, and 14.2 per cent in Scotland.[9] Scotland has always had a higher rate nationally than England and Wales. It is known that the rate of operative delivery is double in British women under the height of 5' 2" (157 cm),[10] but this cannot explain all of the variation between regions. It has been suggested that the higher rate of caesareans in Scotland compared with England

8 Francome, 1990a, p. 81.
9 Savage and Francome, 1993.
10 Chamberlain and Chamberlain, 1975.

is due to the shorter stature of Scottish women. However, McIlwaine, Cole and Macnaughton showed that within Scotland the rate varied from 4.9 to 19.6 per cent in hospitals delivering under 2,000 women; and from 8.7 to 17.4 per cent in hospitals delivering more than that number.[11]

We have found considerable regional variation within England and Wales, and the pattern of this is similar to that found in earlier surveys. The rates in different British hospitals range from 6.2 per cent in one northern district general hospital in a deprived area to 21.5 per cent in an inner-city teaching hospital. This size of difference cannot be justified by differences in case-mix. Women who attend teaching hospitals are more likely to have a caesarean than those in other hospitals.[12]

Regional variations in factors such as height, social class and ethnic mix cannot explain all of the differences in caesarean rates. Some people believe that women should be informed before they book into a hospital for maternity care about the overall rates of intervention and those of individual consultants. After an effective political campaign by women, this is now the law in Massachusetts, in the United States.

In our research, we found that there is no significant correlation between size of hospital, presence or absence of a neonatal intensive care unit, use of epidural anaesthesia, routine electronic fetal monitoring, access to fetal blood sampling equipment, the age or sex of the consultant and the caesarean rate of that obstetrician or hospital. As far as teaching hospitals are concerned, there is also a wide variation in their rates, with the lowest being 10 per cent and the highest 20 per cent.[13]

We did not ask about perinatal mortality rates in our survey of consultants, as these are very dependent on case-mix and transfer policy. However, we compared the caesarean rate for each region with the perinatal mortality rate. If regions with a high caesarean rate had a correspondingly low perinatal mortality rate, this might indicate that these caesareans were saving the lives of babies. However, no such finding occurred.

WHY HAS THE CAESAREAN RATE INCREASED SO MARKEDLY OVER THE LAST TWENTY YEARS IN DEVELOPED COUNTRIES?

Fifty years ago, maternal mortality following caesarean section was much higher than following vaginal delivery, because of infection, thrombosis and anaemia. The improved safety of surgery with modern anaes-

....

11 McIlwaine, Cole and Macnaughton, 1985.
12 Savage and Francome, 1993.
13 Savage and Francome, 1993.

thetic techniques, the availability of antibiotics and of blood transfusion has meant that caesareans are safer than they were. Thus obstetricians, when balancing the risks, have a stronger case for surgery even though there is still a significant maternal mortality and morbidity rate following caesarean section.

There is a second factor which has lowered the threshold for performing the operation in premature labour or in cases of severe high blood pressure (pre-eclampsia) or proven intra-uterine growth retardation on the pre-term infant. This is due to the success of modern neonatal intensive care in saving the lives of low birthweight infants. However, only 1 per cent of births in England and Wales are to babies of 1.5 kg or less, so this factor can explain only a small proportion of the rise in caesarean rates. In a Scottish study, only 1 per cent of births in 1982 were before thirty-two weeks; caesareans in this group accounted for 2.2 per cent of the total caesarean operations, or 0.3 per cent of all deliveries in Scotland in 1982.[14]

The reasons for the rising caesarean rate are complex. Arney, in discussing the way that professional input into birth has developed, calls the present era of obstetrics the 'monitoring' period.[15] He suggests that obstetricians have surrendered their skills to a system of checks and technology. In essence, they have become the slaves of machines, not the masters. There is general agreement in the literature that continuous electronic fetal monitoring in labour of low-risk women increases caesarean rates without significantly improving perinatal mortality rates.[16] Yet electronic fetal monitoring continues to be used indiscriminately on many low-risk women, often without recourse to fetal blood sampling which has been shown to keep caesarean rates down.[17]

Our position is that some increase in the caesarean rate can be justified, but by no means all of the rise that has occurred. There is a great deal of evidence for this position:

• There are wide differences in rates between individual obstetricians. A study of 1,553 affluent low-risk women cared for by eleven obstetricians at a community hospital found an average caesarean rate of 26.9 per cent. However, while one obstetrician had a rate of 19.1 per cent, another had a rate of 42.3 per cent.[18] British evidence shows similar

....

14 McIlwaine et al., 1985.
15 Arney, 1982.
16 Grant in Chalmers, Enkin and Keirse, 1989.
17 MacDonald, Grant, Sheridan-Pereira, Boylan and Chalmers, 1985.
18 Goyert, Bottoms, Treadwell and Nehra, 1989.

variations.[19] Such wide variations could only be explained by personal practice, apparently uninfluenced by current research findings.

• Our evidence shows that many caesareans are conducted because of the fear of litigation in Britain, just as in the United States (see Chapter 8).

• There is evidence of a convenience factor in some places. For example, at one hospital, 9.6 per cent of repeat caesareans occurred at the weekends, when a random distribution would have led to three times that percentage (28.5 per cent) being weekend deliveries.[20]

• There is ample evidence that financial incentives to perform caesareans influence obstetricians' decisions about whether or not to perform a caesarean.[21] Therefore healthier, wealthy women have on average more caesareans than less well-off women.[22]

• Lomas and Enkin state that overall the relative risks and benefits to mother and baby do not appear to be the major factors in the decision to perform a caesarean. They then ask plaintively: 'If the research evidence on the risks, benefits and costs of operative delivery does not determine clinical practice, then what does?'[23]

We have been raising the issue of high caesarean rates since 1978 and are glad to see that some others are beginning to share our view. In 1992, the World Health Organization (WHO) published a report which reviewed the international data and found that countries with high caesarean rates also tended to have the highest level of forceps deliveries. In some countries 'the total proportion of operative deliveries (instrumental + caesarean section) was staggering: approximately one-third of all births in Australia, Greece, Canada and the United States. This finding is almost certainly an indication that a large proportion of interventions are unnecessary or only marginally beneficial'.[24]

In Britain the rates have not risen as high as elsewhere and the evidence shows that the caesarean rate has risen in part because of a move away from forceps deliveries.[25] But again, this can only account for a small part of the rise.

....

19 Francome and Huntingford, 1980.
20 Lomas and Enkin, 1989, p. 1192.
21 Lomas and Enkin, 1989, p. 1191.
22 Taffel et al., 1992, p. 22.
23 Lomas and Enkin, 1989, p. 1189.
24 Stephenson, 1992, p. 28.
25 Francome, 1990b, p. 9.

VAGINAL BIRTH IS STILL SAFER THAN ABDOMINAL DELIVERY

A vaginal birth has always been safer for the mother than a caesarean and this still remains the case. How much of this difference is due to the problem for which the caesarean is performed, and how much is due to the risk of the surgical procedure itself, has been a matter of much debate.

Over the last twenty years, a period for which detailed analysis is available for maternal deaths in England and Wales, the number of maternal deaths fell from 830 in the three years 1964–66 to 163 in the United Kingdom in 1985–87, the last three-year period for which a report has been published. Thus the number of maternal deaths related to the number of births fell from 31.6 to 8.6 per 100,000. During the years 1985–87 there were 76 deaths of women following caesareans. As fewer deaths occurred from 'natural' causes, deaths from caesarean section rose as a proportion from 28.1 to 53.9 per cent of the maternal deaths arising directly from childbirth. The contribution made by caesareans to all maternal deaths rose from 9.8 to 42.3 per cent.[26]

The Confidential Enquiries for 1985–87 show the leading causes of maternal mortality overall in the United Kingdom to have been pulmonary embolism (29 deaths), hypertensive disorders (27), ectopic pregnancy (16), haemorrhage (10), amniotic fluid embolism (9), anaesthesia and sepsis (6 each). The leading causes for deaths caused directly by caesarean section in the United Kingdom were hypertensive disease (14 deaths), pulmonary embolism (9), haemorrhage (5) and anaesthesia (4).

Deaths due to pulmonary embolism are much more likely to follow surgical than vaginal delivery. Pulmonary embolism is difficult to prevent and most fatal cases occur after the woman has left hospital. This suggests that a reduction in surgery could reduce the maternal mortality rate further. The fall in the proportion of all direct deaths following anaesthesia in childbirth from 1.21 per 100,000 in the years 1976–78 to 0.19 per 100,000 in 1985–87 shows the benefits of improvements in anaesthetic technique.

The risks to the mother are higher for an emergency than an elective caesarean. The latest figures show maternal deaths were 0.22 per 100,000 for elective caesareans and 0.5 per 100,000 for emergency caesareans in 1982–84.[27] 'It is unfortunate that no data are available on the numbers of Caesarean sections performed in NHS hospitals in England in this triennium [1985–87] and therefore there is no denomi-

....

26 Department of Health, 1991.
27 Department of Health, 1991.

nator for estimating the fatality rate [from caesareans]'.[28] This has led some obstetricians to plan more elective operations, a trend which would almost certainly increase the caesarean rate still further. Lilford, in a careful analysis of 108 maternal deaths, warned against an uncritical acceptance of this idea.[29] Another reason for not increasing the number of elective compared with emergency operations is that the incidence of respiratory distress syndrome is decreased if the woman has laboured prior to delivery by caesarean.[30]

The Confidential Enquiry reports, 'In 23 cases there was substandard care of direct relevance to the Caesarean section and postoperative management', and concludes, 'An unacceptably high proportion of deaths of women delivered by caesarean section continued to be associated with substandard care. Greater supervision of junior staff and improved facilities for resuscitation are recommended'.[31]

One US study shows that better survival rates following caesareans are possible in one centre of excellence in an urban centre than may be the case nationally, even if the caesarean rates exceed the national rates as was the case here. Frigoletto, Ryan and Philippe reported that at the Boston Women's Hospital 10,231 caesareans were performed in the years 1968–78 without one maternal death directly caused by the operation.[32] The overall maternal mortality rate was 0.72 per 10,000 and the other maternal deaths were early or postpartum and not related to the mode of delivery. The question remains as to whether this can be achieved throughout a country.

In Britain the numbers of maternal deaths are small. Only one obstetrician in ten would be expected to see one maternal death a year. Furthermore, only one in fifty would be likely to see a caesarean-related death in one year, so the risk of caesarean is almost as remote for the individual obstetrician as it is for the individual mother. Although the number of caesarean-related deaths has fallen, the operation is undoubtedly more dangerous for women than a normal vaginal delivery. Thus any further increase in the caesarean rate is likely to lead to the deaths of more women overall.

....

28 Department of Health, 1991, pp. 121–2.
29 Lilford, Van Coeverden De Groot and Moore, 1990.
30 Cohen and Carson, 1985.
31 Department of Health, 1991, p. ix.
32 Frigoletto, Ryan and Phillippe, 1980.

THE STRUCTURE OF THIS BOOK

The next two chapters show the development of the caesarean operation in its historical context and reveal that many current issues were also contentious issues in the past. Some of the practices in the past were somewhat primitive, and we therefore warn pregnant women and other lay readers that they might find some of the material in Chapter 2 disturbing. We then consider the British data in comparison with that of some other countries. In the subsequent two chapters we explain why a caesarean may be necessary and then describe what a woman who needs one might expect from the operation and how she might cope and be best supported afterwards. We then give first-hand information from our survey of women's experiences and what they felt about the operation, whether it was planned or occurred in an emergency. Next, we present the results of our survey of over 300 British obstetricians' views on caesareans. Chapter 9 contains important information about vaginal birth after caesarean and the book concludes with a chapter suggesting constructive ways for women and health professionals to avoid unnecessary caesareans.

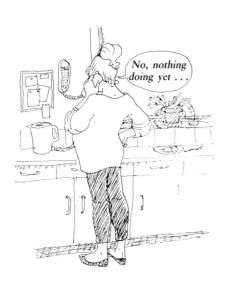

Because some of the information in this book is quite technical, lay readers may choose to begin with Chapters 5, 6 and 10 and Appendix A, before embarking on the rest. It is not necessary for lay readers to understand the statistics in the remainder of the book, but they should feel able to concentrate on those parts of the book most relevant to their needs. Antenatal teachers will, in addition to the above, find much of particular interest to them in Chapter 7.

CHAPTER TWO

THE HISTORY OF CAESAREAN SECTION

As far as the obstetrician facing a difficult labour was concerned, the crucial choice would be what gave the woman the best chance of survival.

THERE are examples of caesareans being carried out in pre-Christian times. Very often the operation would only be performed if the women died during pregnancy: for example, the ancient Hindus only carried out the operation if the mother had died and there were detectable movements of the fetus. There is also some evidence that the operation may have been known to the ancient Egyptians.[1] It is probable that the operation was well known to the early Jews, as it is mentioned in one of the oldest books of Judaism which was first published in pre-Christian times. In fact among this religious group it was carried out on living women who were expected to survive. Their law stated that women having caesareans were not required to observe days of purification as did those who had a vaginal delivery. Such evidence suggests that it is extremely likely that the caesarean section was practised long before the start of the Christian era, although we do not have the history of individual cases.[2] It is quite possible that the skills needed to carry out a successful caesarean were lost over time, for it appears that from early Christian times to the sixteenth century the caesarean section, if it was used at all, was more often practised in cases where the women had died late in pregnancy, in the hope of saving the child.

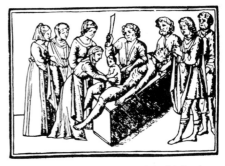

Sixteenth-century depiction of the birth of Julius Caesar

There is debate over the origin of the word 'caesarean'. James Guillimeau said it was 'in imitation of Cesar who was ripped out of his mother's wombe

---

1 Delee, 1913, p. 990.
2 Young, 1944, p. 9.

at the very instant she died'.[3] However, others go back to 715 BC when the king of Rome introduced a law by which it was forbidden to bury a pregnant woman until her child had been removed from her abdomen, even if there was little if any chance of its survival. This was so that the two could be buried separately. Newell suggests that this offers a possible explanation for the origin of the term 'caesarean'. The law, the Lex Regia, became the Lex Cesaria and thus the practice became known as the caesarean operation.[4] However, a totally different and more plausible explanation is proposed by Delee. He suggests that the word comes from the Latin 'cedere' meaning 'to cut' and that the term 'caesarean section' literally means 'cut out'.[5]

THE DEBATE: TO SECTION OR NOT TO SECTION?

Although caesareans came to be usually performed after the death of the woman, it is also likely that throughout history they have been carried out while the woman was still alive but could not deliver vaginally. We shall see from the medical literature that there have been several cases of women carrying out the operation on themselves and it is also likely that there have been many unrecorded cases of women doing this and of those attending them making an attempt to end a long labour. Young suggests that the oldest authentic case of a living child being born by caesarean was that of Georgias, a celebrated orator of Sicily in 508 AD.[6]

However, there are no recorded attempts of performing a caesarean on a living woman in Europe before 1500. Some suggest that this date marks a watershed, for by the sixteenth century claims were being made that a caesarean section with maternal and infant survival was possible. This led to a rethinking of the operation. One school of thought believed that, in the event of obstructed labour, the mother's life could be saved by surgical removal of the child. However, others took the view that chances of survival were so slim that the operation was tantamount to murder. A determined opponent of the operation was Ambrose Pare (1510–90) who condemned those who dared to perform it because 'no man can persuade me [the operation] can be done without the death of the mother'.[7]

In 1581 Rousset wrote an important French paper which opened the debate on the relative benefits of the operation and argued the case for

3 Guillimeau, 1612, p. 185.
4 Newell, 1921, p. 2.
5 Delee, 1913, p. 990.
6 Young, 1944, p. 7.
7 Young, 1944, p. 24.

the possibility of performing a caesarean on a living woman.[8] In fact it was not a medical practitioner but Jacob Nufer, a hog gelder of Sigerhausen, Switzerland, who performed the first recorded successful caesarean section as measured by maternal survival. He carried it out on his wife, Elizabeth Alespachin, during a prolonged and obstructed labour in 1588. Remarkably, reports suggest that both mother and child survived and recovered. Mrs Nufer is said to have gone on to deliver six more children, one set of twins and four single births, and the caesarean child is said to have lived to the age of seventy-seven.[9]

There was a debate on the value of the operation and Guillimeau discussed the usefulness of performing it on a living woman. He did not advocate the practice although he tried it twice, unsuccessfully. 'I know that it may be alleged that there be some have been saved thereby: but though it should happen so, yet ought we rather to admire it rather than practice or imitate it. For "one swallow make not a spring" neither upon one experiment only can one build a science'.[10]

Mercurio became the first surgeon to advocate caesarean section for cases of contracted pelvis in 1604.[11] This suggestion showed that birth attendants had begun to take into account the results of a prenatal examination. Once the decision to carry out a caesarean was taken before labour began, the woman would be in a better physical condition than if she had failed in an attempt at delivery.

On 21 April 1610, Professor Sennert of Wittenberg University recorded a case of a caesarean section being performed by Trautmann on a woman for whom a natural delivery was impossible because of a large hernia.[12] According to Young this operation represents 'The first definitely authentic case of caesarean section intentionally performed upon a living woman'. Unfortunately the woman died twenty-five days after the operation from an infection because the surgeon had not closed the wound or the uterus.[13] Such omission was common. According to accounts at the time, during the sixteenth and seventeenth centuries the caesarean operation was very rudimentary. Anaesthetics were unknown and the patient was tied down or held by assistants. The wound was not stitched but left gaping. Attempts were occasionally made to bring

8 Young, 1944, p. 23.
9 Hull, 1798, p. 38.
10 Guillimeau, 1612, p. 187.
11 Young, 1944, p. 28.
12 Newell, 1921, p. 4.
13 Young, 1944, p. 30.

the abdominal walls together by a couple of crude stitches, bandages and/or sticking plaster.[14]

Performing the operation on a living woman therefore remained highly controversial. In 1616 William Harvey, renowned for discovering the circulation of the blood, was one of those who took the view that the caesarean operation should only be used on the death of the mother.[15]

THE ROLE OF THE CHURCH

During pre-industrial times religion played a leading role in the decision-making of most aspects of life, including pregnancy and childbirth. The Catholic Church banned abortions if the fetus was forty-four days old in the case of a male and eighty-eight days in the case of a female, and from 1869 it proscribed abortion throughout pregnancy.

In 1733 the medical profession asked the doctors of theology at the Sorbonne whether it was religiously correct to sacrifice the woman in order to try to save the life of the baby in the case where a woman could not deliver vaginally. On 30 March they replied that if one could only save the life of one or the other, there was a conflict. Justice would imply that it was better to sacrifice the baby. However, they believed that, according to charity, it was better to save the baby because it was only at the expense of the mother's own life that the baptism of the child could be assured and eternal life therefore secured.[16] This ruling meant that craniotomy (the perforation, breaking or crushing of the fetal skull) in order to save the life of the mother was not allowable. It was their view that the child must be removed in order that it might be baptised. This would save it from having to spend eternity in 'Limbo', a place which, according to the official doctrines of the Church, was between heaven and hell. In fact, other Church authorities have in the past suggested an even worse fate. As late as 22 May 1936 the major Catholic paper *The Universe* stated: 'It is now, and always has been, the mind of the Church that unbaptised infants go to hell.'

The Church also advocated a caesarean in a case where the woman had died. This is similar to the earliest practices in ancient civilisations, but the justification was different. The rationale of the Catholic Church was that a caesarean might save the soul of the child. Guillimeau stressed the importance of the operation 'that thereby the child may be saved and receive baptism'.[17] He continued:

....

14 Young, 1944, p. 33.
15 Young, 1944, p. 38.
16 Young, 1944, p. 41.
17 Guillimeau, 1612, p. 224.

Lawyers judge them worthy of death, who shall bury a great bellied woman that is dead before the child is taken forth because they seem to destroy the hope of a living creature. The chirurgion must be certainly assured that the woman is dead, and that her kinsfolk, friends and others that are present, do all affirm that her soul is departed.[18]

He proposed that, to be assured that the mother had in fact died, one should place some light feathers over her mouth for with even light breath they would fly away.[19]

In fact the practice of carrying out a caesarean if the mother had died carried on right up until the 1930s. In the fifth edition of his book *Moral Problems in Hospital Practice*, published in 1935, Finney stated:

The canon directs that, if the mother dies during pregnancy, the fetus should be extracted by those upon whom this duty devolves . . . the Catholic physician is obliged to perform the caesarean operation in all stages of pregnancy beginning with the period when the embryo is distinguishable and has the form of a fetus . . . This fourth provision of the canon is based on the fact that the fetus often survives the mother who dies after delivery and therefore nothing should be left undone to extract the fetus without delay, because, under the circumstances there is nearly always the chance to administer baptism and therefore secure eternal life for the fetus.[20]

In his book Finney stresses the importance of ensuring that the woman is in fact dead prior to the performance of the operation, as in some cases the woman had been killed by this kind of intervention.[21] Baudelocque related a case in which a birth attendant thought a woman had died and extracted the child.[22] The woman, who had apparently fainted, woke up and complained of the injury done to her and the surgeon fled. They had difficulty in persuading him to return to sew up the wound. Fortunately the woman recovered but, unfortunately for the surgeon, she developed a hernia and sued, arguing that the wrong kind of needle had been used.

It does not seem that post-mortem caesarean was often successful,

18 Guillimeau, 1612, p. 185.
19 Guillimeau, 1612, p. 186.
20 Finney, 1935, p. 46.
21 Finney, 1935, p. 46.
22 Baudelocque, 1801.

although extravagant claims were sometimes made. Hyman and Lange reported 331 cases during the nineteenth century up to 1878 when only nineteen children were saved.[23]

CAESAREANS IN THE EIGHTEENTH CENTURY

From the early eighteenth century, doctors became increasingly involved in obstetric practice with a resultant increase in publications on the subject. The numbers of caesareans being performed slowly increased and successful cases were described in great detail, success still being measured in terms of maternal survival. Some earlier attempts had managed to save the child but had resulted in maternal death.

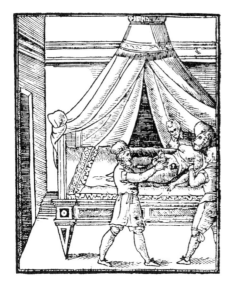

The operation was more commonly performed on the Catholic continent and, in part because it was less often the last resort, it had more success than in Britain. It was still controversial and rather dangerous for the women involved. Writing in 1788, Jaques René Tenon recorded only seventy-nine successful caesarean sections in the whole of Europe since 1500.[24]

The first *recorded* caesarean section performed in Great Britain was by Smith, an Edinburgh surgeon, on 29 June 1737, when summoned to a woman who had been in labour for six days. On examination he found that a normal delivery was impossible and performed the caesarean section with the approval of two other physicians and the relatives of the patient who had been warned of the risks involved. Unfortunately the child was removed dead and the woman died the following day.[25]

In the following year, the first successful caesarean section in the United Kingdom was recorded. It was performed by a midwife, Mary Donally, and the mother was Alice O'Neale, aged 33, a farmer's wife

....

23 Young, 1944, p. 229.
24 Young, 1944, p. 50.
25 Young, 1944, p. 36.

of Charlemont, Ireland, who was the mother of several children. Alice had been in labour for twelve days, numerous midwives had attended her and attempted treatment but with no success. The child was believed to be dead after the third day. In desperation they called in Donally, a local woman famous among the community for extracting dead births. After trying to deliver the patient without success she performed a caesarean operation. On removing the dead infant Mary Donally held the sides of the wound together with her hands while neighbours went to fetch silk and a tailor's needle with which she stitched the wound. Alice O'Neale made a full recovery but later developed a large ventral hernia (as did many other patients of caesarean section at that time). Donally smeared the wound with the white of eggs. Duncan Stewart, a surgeon from Dungannon, wrote:

> In about twenty seven days the patient was able to walk a mile on foot, and came to me in a farmer's house, where she showed me the wound covered with a cicatrice, but she complained of her belly hanging outwards on the right side where I . . . advised to support the side of her belly with a bandage. The patient has enjoyed good health ever since, manages her family affairs, and has frequently walked to market in this town which is six miles distance from her own house.[26]

The fact that the first successful operation was done by a midwife did not please the medical profession and in the literature there was much disparagement of midwife Donally's success. As late as 1944, Young called the achievement 'a matter of good luck rather than good judgement'.[27]

It was not until 1793 that the first successful British caesarean performed by a physician was carried out. James Barlow, a surgeon of Blackburn, Lancashire, was tending Jane Foster who had an extremely deformed pelvis due to being run over by a loaded cart prior to becoming pregnant. When she went 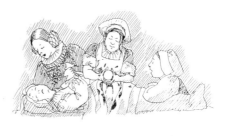 into labour she understandably became very distressed and was in much

26 Stewart, 1747, pp. 361–2.
27 Young, 1944, p. 54.

pain. As normal delivery was impossible, caesarean section was suggested and the likely outcome of the operation explained to the patient. Her pain and distress being considerable by this time, Mrs Foster agreed with little hesitation. The operation was performed with no anaesthetic, the wound was stitched and the patient was then wrapped in flannel. While the mother survived, the child died.[28] During the rest of the century, however, six further attempts at caesareans failed and Radford recorded that in Britain at the end of the eighteenth century there had been nineteen caesarean section operations and only two mothers and seven children had survived. However, he was of the opinion that this figure was remarkable considering that the operation was such a 'hazardous undertaking' at that time.[29]

The first successful caesarean performed in the United States was carried out by Dr Jesse Bennet on his own wife in 1794 in a frontier settlement in the Shenandoah Valley in Virginia. Labour was difficult owing to a contracted pelvis and Dr Alex Humphrey was called for consultation. Forceps failed and the wife did not want a craniotomy. Dr Humphrey would not perform the caesarean and so Dr Bennet did it himself. His wife was stretched out on a crude plank resting on two barrels and put under the influence of a large dose of opium. The *Journal of the American Medical Association* (vol. 115, p. 1940) stated dramatically: 'The courageous frontier surgeon by one quick stroke of the knife opened the abdomen and uterus and quickly delivered the child and placenta. At this stage he delayed long enough to remove the ovaries. The wounds were closed by a stout linen thread and contrary to the expectations of everyone present Mrs Bennet was soon well and active.'

The baby daughter lived to be seventy-seven, so there were some successes with the operation. However, before 1800 caesarean sections had largely been 'operations of desperation', performed as a last resort on dying mothers, in an attempt to save the baby. Those British surgeons who dared to perform it were most often treated with scorn and condemnation by their colleagues, so that few would actually attempt the operation.

One important point is that the women undergoing the operation were usually in a very bad physical condition. The length of labour before the operation is known in fourteen of the nineteen recorded cases. All but two had been in labour for longer than thirty hours, and four had laboured for a period of over five days.

....

28 Young, 1944, p. 54.
29 Radford, 1865, p. 11.

Symphyseotomy as an alternative to caesarean During the eighteenth century, surgeons began to experiment with other forms of surgical intervention to aid labour. Thus in 1777, the poor success rate of the caesarean operation meant that it was almost entirely superseded by the development of a new operative delivery technique.[30] The symphyseotomy operation was introduced by a French surgeon, M. Sigault. His earlier proposal for the operation, in which he suggested that it should be tested on animals and condemned criminals, was not favourably received. The later proposal, which was successfully tested on a patient, consisted of cutting through the skin in the direction of the pubic bone and then dividing the junction of the cartilaginous symphysis with the knife. The knees of the patient which were being held firmly by assistants could then be gently forced apart in order to separate the bones, thus making room for the delivery of the child under the strength of the uterine contractions. If this failed, embryotomy was performed. 'The section of the symphysis pubis, it was thought, would banish for ever the use of crotchets, or perforators and other destructive instruments, as well as premature delivery and the cesarean operation'.[31]

Subsequent to his initial attempt, Sigault operated on four other women, one of whom died. Although Sigault was the first to propose and successfully perform the operation, it was M. Le Roy, an assistant at the operation, who was the first to publish an account of it. However, opposition to the operation was strong. In 1803, Hamilton wrote: 'from the history of between 30 and 40 cases, where the division of the symphysis pubis was performed on the continent, and one case in Great Britain, we consider ourselves authorised to condemn that operation in every view, and advise that it be had recourse to *in no case whatever*'.[32]

As time went on, Sigault became less confident about the procedure and before his death he recommended caesarean section instead of symphyseotomy for difficult deliveries. The operation still continues to be used in some countries and the Maternity Report of St Luke's Hospital, Anua, Nigeria, reveals that in 1991 a total of twenty symphyseotomy operations were carried out.

The debate over caesareans in Britain and France The year 1798 was very important in deciding the future of policy for performing caesareans during the nineteenth

....

30 Newell, 1921, p. 5.
31 Baudelocque, 1801, pp. 48–9.
32 Hamilton, 1803, p. 333.

century. This ended with doctors in Britain and France making different decisions about the operation.

In France Baudelocque presented a report to the Society of Medicine in Paris, in September 1798. In it he said that the caesarean operation was once again the subject of great controversy. He admitted that the operation was not always successful but supported it and argued that if the caesarean was not performed the woman's fate would often be worse than death.[33] He pointed out that the vaginal birth of a child alive is generally impossible when the diameter of the pelvis is only 2½ inches. He considered craniotomy to be very dangerous for the woman and also that one should not kill the child.[34] He gave notes of seventy-three cases, of which thirty-one mothers survived and where the main indication for the operation was a distortion of the pelvis. He continued to argue: 'Far from prohibiting the caesarean operation, other laws should oblige us to perform it, if we can demonstrate that this operation is the only one which can preserve the child without being essentially fatal to the mother.'

After a discussion of Baudelocque's report the Society of Medicine accepted that the operation had been a success and in some cases could lead to saving the lives of both the mother and baby. It unanimously decided that it was the duty of the physician to carry out caesareans and that 200 extra copies of Baudelocque's report should be sent to different judicial and administrative bodies.[35] There was some opposition outside the Society, notably from a colourful character called Saccombe who had studied in England under William Hunter, the best known of the contemporary British obstetricians. He called Baudelocque a 'murderer' for one of his patients had died after a caesarean and claimed that he himself could deliver any woman with his hands. In 1798 he formed his 'Ecole Anti-Caesarienne' but was fined 3,000 francs for the slander of Baudelocque and fled the country.

Three months after the decision in Paris, the Manchester obstetrician W. Simmons wrote his 'Reflection on the Propriety of Performing the Caesarean Operation' in which he ignored the two successful cases and argued that, in contrast to the rest of Europe, the operation was universally fatal in England.[36] Believing the rates for other countries to be of no relevance, he therefore advocated the traditional conservative use of

....

33 Baudelocque, 1801, p. 14.
34 Baudelocque, 1801, p.37.
35 Baudelocque, 1801, p.101.
36 Simmons, 1799.

the operation only in the event of the death of the mother. He also quoted Hunter's view that the life of the woman was more important than that of the fetus. He recommended the use of craniotomy and stated: 'the child may be extracted by the crochet whatever the distortion shall be, if in any part of the cavity there shall be a space of 1½" in diameter'.[37] The normal range in Britain today is 4"–5¾" (10–14 cm), with an average of 5" (12 cm).

This opened up an acrimonious debate. Hull, a fellow Mancunian, took exception to Simmons's condemnation of caesarean section. In a reply written in a paper published later that month he pointed out many discrepancies in Simmons's argument against the operation, not least his assertion that it is always fatal to the mother. He also argued that there could never be a pelvis so contracted that at some point there was not 1½" diameter.[38]

Hull's book, entitled *A Defence of the Caesarean Operation*, questioned whether the operation was always fatal to the mother and listed the situations in which he would recommend the use of the operation:

1. Where the Mother is dead, for the preservation of her Offspring;
2. Where the Child is dead, or supposed to be so, for the preservation of the Parent;
3. Where the Mother and Child are living, for the preservation of both.[39]

Hull quoted Simmons as saying that the caesarean 'has proved fatal in England in every instance' and is 'an operation that has proved so fatal to my country women' that it must be abandoned.[40] He went to great lengths to point out the difference between the patient 'dying *from an operation*, and *after an operation*'.[41] Hull went on to accuse Simmons of being 'blinded by prejudice' and suggested that he had made his judgement on cases without knowledge of the full facts and conditions of the patient in each case, and as such 'the value of the operation ought to be appreciated' for certain cases.[42]

Simmons responded to Hull's work following the death of a woman, Elizabeth Thompson, in Manchester after a caesarean operation. The

....

[37] Young, 1944, p. 60.
[38] Hull, 1798, pp. 5–7.
[39] Hull, 1798, p. 5.
[40] Simmons, 1799, p. 30, quoted in ibid., p. 7.
[41] Hull, 1798, p. 8, emphasis in original.
[42] Hull, 1798, pp. 8–10.

theme of Simmons's response was that to perform the operation on a living woman was tantamount to murder. Throughout his writings Simmons upheld the notion that only God is able to decide who should live and who should die.[43]

The debate that took place between Hull and Simmons is an important one in the history of caesarean section because it highlighted the relative advantages and disadvantages of performing the operation. As Radford states, the controversy 'brought the greater part of the medical profession to entertain more clear and definite opinions'.[44] However, the balance of the view in Britain, contrary to that in France, was against the operation.

Baudelocque made an influential contribution to the caesarean section debate in his *Two Memoirs on the Cesarean Operation* (1798 and 1799), (translated by Hull in 1801). While accepting the necessity of the operation for contracted pelvis and other unusual conditions, Baudelocque added the condition of tumours of the vagina as an indication. He therefore highlighted the fact that there are some cases where vaginal delivery is absolutely impossible and caesarean section was thus the only option available to extract the fetus. Baudelocque was critical of other interventionist techniques such as the use of the crochet, symphyseotomy and induction, suggesting that laws needed to be passed obliging obstetricians to carry out caesarean section in certain circumstances, rather than outlawing its practice as some of his predecessors had argued.[45]

In Britain the anti-caesarean school was in the ascendant and led to the difference in practice from the rest of Europe.

CAESAREANS IN THE NINETEENTH CENTURY

At the beginning of the nineteenth century the bulk of British obstetric opinion was opposed to caesareans and the textbooks of the time reflected that view. Alexander Hamilton, for example, published one entitled *Outlines of the Theory and Practice of Midwifery* in which he argued against the indications commonly used to justify the operation: 'Experience has proved, that where ready access is obtained for the admission of the necessary instruments, the head of the child may, by the operation of embryotomy, be so diminished . . . [that] the extraction of the mangled infant is practicable'[46]

....

43 Simmons, 1799, p. 231.
44 Radford, 1865, p. 1.
45 Baudelocque, 1801, p. 9.
46 Hamilton, 1803, pp. 270–1.

He gives great detail of particular cases, charting every stage of complicated labours, including one case of a woman with extreme contraction of the pelvis where the pelvic gap was so narrow that Hamilton's instruments could not be introduced into the uterus in order to extract the child. Despite the fact that the woman died after great suffering, Hamilton went on to state: 'the histories of the [caesarean] operation, hitherto on record, do not appear to me to contain the ample information which would be required by one compelled to perform it'[47]

A royal catastrophe   A catastrophic royal birth in 1817 appears to have been the catalyst for more caesarean sections in this country. Sir Richard Croft attended Princess Charlotte and allowed an obstructed labour to continue in preference to using forceps or dismembering the heir to the throne of England. Fearing her death from caesarean section, Sir Richard did nothing. The infant was stillborn, the princess died, and three months later Sir Richard shot himself.[48] These events had a major historical impact. They brought Queen Victoria to the throne and marked an important turning point away from 'ultra-conservatism' in obstetrics.

Saving the women   British obstetricians were often critical of their European counterparts for carrying out caesareans unnecessarily. A French doctor in 1829 commented that when the smallest diameter of the pelvis was nearly 2¼ inches, the child must be alive and the decision had to be taken whether to follow the English and destroy the fetus or, on the other hand, to give it life while exposing the mother to great danger. The French generally took the latter position while an unnamed English doctor commented, 'Pity the poor French women we say'. However, it would be wrong to assume that the French doctors never performed embryotomy, for in 1849 several cases were reported where it was tried before a caesarean was performed.[49]

In Britain the preconditions for a caesarean were strict and, after reviewing the evidence of the years 1822–62, Young commented: 'The highest authorities in Great Britain at this time fixed the degree of pelvic contraction in which the dimensions varied from 3–3½ inches in the long diameter as the lowest limit below which delivery by embryotomy could be performed' and below which it was always necessary to perform a

....

47 Hamilton, 1803, p. 293.
48 National Institutes of Health, 1982, p. 52.
49 Young, 1944, pp. 74–8.

caesarean.[50] Instead there were three other major methods in the case of a difficult delivery.

The alternatives to caesarean

Forceps

Forceps were in popular use as an aid to difficult deliveries during the nineteenth century. Once again there were proponents on both sides of the debate. For example, Radford claims that:

> This instrument most justly takes a high position in obstetrics, because its sole employment is for the preservation of life. It is intended, within a certain range of protracted labour, to supersede craniotomy. In the hands of a discreet and judicious practitioner, it is both a safe and a very powerful instrument. Before its introduction into practice, whenever turning could not be performed, the child was doomed to destruction by craniotomy.[51]

Further, Radford stated that 'There are no statistics published which afford any truthful information either as to the frequency of the application of this instrument, or as to the mortality of those women who have been delivered by it'.[52] He claimed that he had used forceps many times and never had a death as a result of their application.

The debate over the relative benefits of forceps as opposed to caesarean section still continues in the twentieth century and the latest evidence shows that the use of forceps has diminished as caesareans have become safer.[53]

Craniotomy

This is a difficult and upsetting procedure by which the head is crushed in the womb in order to make it small enough to pass through the vaginal canal. The procedure was a very difficult one as may be seen by some of the recorded case histories. J. Hamilton, for example, described in 1840 how, in a woman with width at the pelvic brim of only 1½ inches,

....

50 Young, 1944, p. 76.
51 Radford, 1865, p. 27.
52 Radford, 1865, p. 29.
53 Francome, 1990b, p. 13,

he performed a craniotomy at midnight but did not completely finish with his efforts until 2.00 the next afternoon. The woman was saved and he was 'carried home in a sedan chair exhausted'.[54]

If the head was not the part of the body presenting then the operation was called an embryotomy and there was continuing debate about the rectitude of killing the child about to be delivered. Many argued that it had no sensation of feeling or pain.[55] However, the procedure was difficult and the obstetrician had to gather all the pieces together to make sure that nothing had been left inside the woman. There were strong critics. Bedford stated in 1844: 'The man who would wantonly thrust an instrument of death into the brain of a living foetus, would not scruple, under the mantle of night, to use the stilleto of the assassin'.[56]

Churchill in 1855 gave the mortality rate of craniotomy as about one in five. He also said that in Britain the operation occurred once in 219 deliveries compared to once in 1,205 deliveries in France, and was even more rare in Germany with one in 1,944 deliveries. To make a comparison he collected data for 321 operations since 1750 and said that the majority of women (172) had died. In 1872 Parry pointed out that the overall death rate of one in five masked the fact that women with a width at the pelvic brim of 2½ inches or below had a death rate of 38 per cent.[57] However, even such analysis did not undermine the essential fact that, at that time, maternal mortality was lower for a craniotomy than for a caesarean and was therefore the preferable British policy unless one gave high value to the fetus.

In Catholic countries theologians often gave the fetus a very high status and, as doctrine has changed so much in recent years, it is important to remember the official doctrine of the time. As late as 1935 papal authority approved the publication in London and St Louis of the fifth edition of the book *Moral Problems in Hospital Practice*. It stated:

> To preserve one's life is generally speaking duty; but it may be the plainest duty, the highest duty, to sacrifice one's life. War is full of such instances, in which it is not man's duty to live but to die . . . a parallel case, is the situation of a woman in a difficult labour, when her life and that of her unborn child are in extreme danger. In this situation it is the mother's duty to die rather than to consent to the killing of her child.

....
54 Young, 1944, p. 77.
55 Young, 1944, p. 79.
56 Young, 1944, p. 80.
57 Young, 1944, p. 82.

The author Patrick Finney continued: 'The first fact in the world is that justice, law and order should be observed no matter what the cost; better that ten thousand mothers should die than one foetus be unjustly killed'.[58]

Finney's book was reviewed in the British medical literature and widely read. He balanced the life of one fetus with ten thousand women. Others went even further. A. J. Shulte, a professor of liturgy, stated: 'Even if the life of the mother is in danger, a physician has no right to destroy the child's life. I say now and with all seriousness that it is better that one million mothers die than to have one innocent little creature killed.'[59]

With such attitudes it is clear that strict Catholic doctors, nurses and mothers would not agree with craniotomy.

Despite the dominant British view being in favour of craniotomy ther were a few in Britain who also became concerned with the loss of fet; life. In 1865 Radford calculated, on the evidence available to him, tha 2,861 infants were being destroyed annually by this operation and sug gested that this figure was an extremely conservative estimate.[60]

A determined opponent of craniotomy, Radford argued that if craniotomy was used, certain great men (sic) would not have been born – an argument that was to be repeated later by opponents of birth control: 'Suppose the head of Shakespeare had been opened, what would have been the loss to society.' In addition he commented: 'It is one thing to deliver the woman, and another to do so safely. It is much to be deplored, that this operation is still permitted to be so unconditionally performed'.[61]

However, this minority view did not hold much appeal, and the clear view among British obstetricians was that caesarean was such a dangerous operation that it must be the last resort.

Induction

Induction of premature labour was not originally intended to supersede caesarean section but rather to prevent craniotomy.[62] If a woman had endured a craniotomy at full term and again fell pregnant, she could then have earlier induction of labour with much greater safety. The state of contraception was so bad that one woman who could not deliver

....

58 Finney, 1935.
59 Shulte, 1917.
60 Radford, 1865, pp. 44–5.
61 Radford, 1865, p. 48; Francome, 1984, p. 59.
62 Radford, 1865, p. 35.

normally had eleven pregnancies between 1862 and 1885. Eight of these ended in embryotomy and in three others labour was induced halfway through pregnancy.[63]

However, according to Radford, in general, by the time induction of labour was proposed, the woman had passed the period when a caesarean could be advantageously performed. Radford objected to this situation, stating that induction was not as safe a technique as was commonly presented, and indeed sometimes caused the death of the mother;[64] he advocated caesarean section instead.

As far as the obstetrician facing a difficult labour was concerned, the crucial choice would be what gave the woman the best chance of survival.

Safety of caesareans until the 1870s

After the first successful caesarean in England there were six other caesareans in which the mother died, until the second successful one was performed in April 1834, nearly forty years later.[65] Radford stated that 'The statistics of the results of the caesarean section, especially as concerns the mothers, are highly unfavourable.' He recorded that, of seventy-seven British and Irish women whose cases were tabled, sixty-six (86 per cent) died and eleven (14 per cent) survived. From those seventy-seven cases, seventy-eight infants were extracted (including one case of twins), forty-six (59 per cent) of the infants survived and thirty-two (41 per cent) died. Radford claimed that nearly all of the infants that did not survive were dead before the operation and it was his opinion that the infants might have been saved if the caesarean section had been performed earlier.[66]

One of the best pieces of research into mortality was that of Kayser of Copenhagen. He suggested that there were many cases that were not reported, but that of the 338 operations on record from 1750 to 1839, 38 per cent of women survived. He felt that this was an overestimate because in 67 cases in which the operation was carried out in a hospital, where concealment would be much more difficult, the success rate was only 20 per cent and he believed care would have been better than average. He may have been wrong, of course, because infections were likely to be much more common in hospitals. However, one of his findings was that the success rate was improving. During the period 1750–1800 one-third of women survived (32 per cent); from 1801 to 1832 37

63 Young, 1944, p. 144.
64 Radford, 1865, pp. 42–3.
65 Young, 1944, p. 58.
66 Radford, 1865, p. 7.

per cent survived; and from 1833–1839 over half (51 per cent) survived. He also found that where the woman had been in labour for seventy-two hours or more, the success rate was only 28 per cent, whereas if labour was under twenty-four hours the success rate was four out of five (80 per cent).[67]

Table 2.1   *Some international rates of caesarean survival 1800–80*

Country	Period	Number of cases	% mothers survived	Source
USA	To 1877	80	48	Young (1944)
Germany	To 1872	712	47	Schroeder (1873)
France	To 1872	344	45	Schroeder (1873)
Britain	To 1879	131	18	Radford (1880)

The results show that survival rates in Britain were below half of those in the other three countries. This difference had been known throughout the nineteenth century although it had not been so clearly documented before, and in 1833 Campbell pointed out that this difference was at least in part due to the fact that on the continent the operation was carried out in different circumstances. First, they often performed it when in Britain it would not have been carried out at all; and second, it was carried out earlier in the pregnancy. Other later obstetricians held a similar view.[68] However, in making comparison with the United States, Harris declared that the major reason was the poor state of the British women when they came to have the operation. They had poor nutrition and drank too much. It is, however, unlikely that the British women drank more than the French and so this is unlikely to be the real reason.

By the middle of the nineteenth century the British were taking a slightly more positive view towards caesareans. It was the influence of Radford among the medical profession that began the shift in position towards a more accepting climate for the operation.[69] Even so it was only performed occasionally on a living woman. This was usually when a craniotomy could not be performed: if, for example, ovarian cysts prevented access to the fetus. In other words, it would only be performed when everything else had been tried and had failed.[70]

....

67 Young, 1944, p. 87.
68 Young, 1944, pp. 88–91.
69 Young, 1944, p. 75.
70 Newell, 1921, p. 3.

'SISTERS WERE DOING IT FOR THEMSELVES!'

Throughout history, many women have performed the caesarean operation on themselves. Presumably ignorant of any surgical procedure, these operations were performed out of fear and desperation. In the majority of such cases the outcome was not good for the infant. Often the child would die before or during the complicated labour, or else it would die due to mutilation from the surgery.

The earliest known case of a woman performing the operation on herself was recorded in 1769 in the West Indies. It was suggested that the woman had carried out the operation because of impatience with the pain of a prolonged labour,[71] although, of course, this explanation is that of an observer and not of the woman herself.

The first recorded case in the United States was on 29 January 1822, when a 14-year-old girl performed the operation on herself. She was carrying twins and delivered herself lying in a snowbank. After delivery of the first baby she buried it in the snow. Doctors were called in to remove the second child and to attend to the wound. The patient survived but the fate of the other child is unknown.[72]

In 1876 Von Guggenberg reported that a woman in labour for three days performed a caesarean section, which she had heard was possible, on herself to obtain relief from abdominal distention and violent pain. The child did not survive although it is possible that it was dead before the operation as the mother reported that fetal movements had ceased. Her wound was treated by a physician and she made a full recovery.[73]

In Turkey, in 1879, a woman cut open her abdomen and uterus with a razor after being in labour for over thirty-six hours without progressing. The wound was then sewn up by a neighbour and both mother and child apparently survived.[74] The fact that the operation was considered so dangerous meant that the case of an Italian woman carrying out a caesarean on herself created a great deal of surprise in 1886. A 23-year-old single woman, seven months pregnant, was talked about and faced a great deal of questioning from her family as to the reasons for her increase in weight. Fearing the shame, she cut open her abdomen with a sharp carving knife and brought out the baby in pieces. In the evening she took a cloth soaked in blood a few miles to her sister's house to 'prove' that she had menstruated. Her subsequent illness led to medical

71 Baudelocque, 1801, p. 66.
72 Young, 1944, p. 13.
73 Young, 1944, p. 14.
74 Young, 1944, p. 13.

attention and the operation being noted in the medical records. *The Lancet* wrote to the doctors involved in the case and received confirmation and further details.[75]

Interestingly it appears that women 'doing it for themselves' at this time was actually safer than the so-called professional procedures. An American medical historian, R. P. Harris, recorded a 66 per cent survival and recovery rate for women performing the operation on themselves compared to a rate of 37.5 per cent for American physicians up to 1888, and 14 per cent for their British counterparts.[76] This is possible considering that the woman was more likely than the hospital surgeon to be using clean implements and was less likely to be using equipment that had just been used to carry out a post-mortem or to perform surgery on a patient with a fatal infection. However, also important was that the women who carried out the operation on themselves were on average in better physical shape than the women being given a caesarean after all else had failed. Furthermore, the unusual case of a successful caesarean was more likely to be reported to the medical journals than an unsuccessful one.

NEW AGE OF CAESAREANS

The dangers of the operation meant that in Britain the caesarean was usually only carried out when a craniotomy could not be performed, possibly because ovarian cysts prevented access to the fetus. An example of this is provided by a debate in *The Lancet* in 1881. In the June edition, a Dr John Galton described a caesarean where a patient died. In the July edition he was attacked by A. C. Tweedie (25 June): 'It seems a somewhat new thing for this very formidable operation to be at all warranted where there is no pelvic deformity. I am satisfied that had I a similar case to deal with I would be able to accomplish delivery without having recourse to caesarean section.' However, Galton retorted that although he had not specifically stated it in his paper, the description of the symptoms should have alerted Tweedie to the fact that the woman had cancer and that caesarean section is indicated where there is malignant disease of the lower segment of the uterus.

In the 1880s there were new developments of technique which changed the balance of risks of the operation and led to it becoming safer than craniotomy *for women who were relatively early on in labour*. This was due to a number of improvements in general medical practice, including

75 Baliva and Serpierri, 1886, pp. 890 and 994.
76 Young, 1944, p. 17.

the introduction of the sterilisation of instruments, the use of anaesthetics and also specific improvements in technique.

A major change began in 1876, when Porro of Pavia developed his technique. In his own city no woman had ever survived the operation. Porro carried out a caesarean on a young woman with a distorted pelvis due to rickets. The child lived but the mother died fifty hours later from haemorrhage and peritonitis. It appeared to him that the greatest risk to the woman came from the damaged uterus. The incision in the uterine walls allowed the escape of infected lochia into the pelvic cavity. He therefore advised amputation of the body of the uterus in order to lessen the dangers of haemorrhage and infection. The wound surface of the uterine stump would be much smaller than that of the whole uterus and he knew it was easier to control the haemorrhage from his experience of previous operations to remove ovarian tumours. Porro carried out the first successful operation on 21 May 1876. The woman had been under observation for twenty-four days and the operation was carried out seven hours into labour. Porro and his assistants washed their hands in a dilute solution of carbolic acid and administered chloroform. The child also survived.

When others tried the operation the results at first were mixed. In fact, the next three women all died but two children lived. Three out of the first four women operated on in the United States died, and four out of the first five in Britain. However, some places showed a remarkable improvement and none greater than the Vienna lying-in hospital. Here, in the previous one hundred years not a single woman had recovered. From 1877 to 1885 there were twenty-seven Porro operations with nearly half (48 per cent) of the women surviving. Then in the following three years there was a remarkable series of operations and out of twenty-seven cases, all except two of the women lived.[77]

Harris advanced a number of reasons for the improved results of the Porro operation, which included the following:

- Carrying it out electively and not as the last resort.
- Operating early in labour.
- Rigorous antiseptic technique.
- Washing all the blood out of the abdominal cavity.
- Antiseptic treatment of the stump of the uterus.

Harris said that, at that time (in 1880), there was only an average of about three caesareans a year in the United States, many women died

[77] Newell, 1921, p. 5.

undelivered and that to increase the number by the Porro operation might be helpful to women.[78] In a second article in the same year he collated the results of the first fifty Porro operations carried out in Europe, in which twenty-one women and forty-three children were saved.[79]

There was some opposition to the operation on the grounds that it sterilised the woman. One of the most vehement was in the *American Journal of Obstetrics* in 1883, where Schlemmer argued that the oper-ation was against religious tenets and that men should not have marital intercourse with wives who had undergone it.[80] This advice was easier to give than to receive. In contrast, the English writer Dr Playfair said that many women needing caesareans suffered from rickets and came from the poorer parts of the community suffering from ill-nourishment.[81] He continued by suggesting that the sterilisation may have been of benefit to the community. Others prophetically saw Porro's method as a transi-tory one and this is what it became.

The caesarean operation was revolutionised in 1882 by the German Max Sanger (1853–1903). He publicised his results in the *American Journal of Obstetrics* in 1886. Sanger believed that any operation to replace craniotomy needed to save not only the woman and child but also the reproductive organs. Others had experimented with suturing the uterus and in the 1870s this technique seemed to become more widely used. Braxton Hicks used silver wire, as did Robert Barnes. However, Sanger proposed many more sutures than had been used hitherto and a procedure of closing the uterus in layers by the use of sutures or stitches. This would 'close the uterine wound by a system of deep (muscular) and superficial (peritoneal) sutures and so keep the uterine and peritoneal cavities shut off' (*The Lancet*, April 1891, p. 885). The eight or ten deep sutures were made of silver and about twenty superficial ones of silk. The advantage of so many sutures was that each one had to bear less strain and so was unlikely to break. At previous autopsies a gaping wound had often been found.

Sanger did not make any grand claims about having invented a new method of operating. Rather, he painstakingly studied the developments and innovations of the operation, comparing success rates, and came to a conclusion which brought together the best of what had gone before.[82]

....
78 Harris, 1980a, p. 356.
79 Harris, 1980b, p. 134.
80 Young, 1944, p. 104.
81 Playfair, 1886.
82 Young, 1944, p. 136.

The first operation carried out according to Sanger's recommendations was done by G. Leopold in Leipzig on 25 May 1882 and the mother and child made a smooth recovery. However, the next two operations were not successful. It is surprising that Sanger himself did not carry out the operation according to his own suggestions until 4 December 1884 when it was the tenth to be performed. The mother and child made a good recovery.

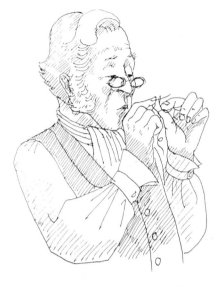

Analysis of the first fifty Sanger operations by Harris in the United States up to 1887 showed that 70 per cent were saved, compared to only 40 per cent of the first fifty Porro operations.[83] Closer analysis of the data showed that of the first fifty operations, thirty-three were done in Germany: all but one of the children and all but four of the mothers were saved. However, in seventeen operations carried out abroad, only six mothers were saved. This may be in part because, in Germany, the criteria for performing the operation had been relaxed, but it is probably also indicative of greater experience and skill.

Some information that caesareans might be becoming safer was published in *The Lancet* (6 January 1886). Dr Playfair referred to the statistics of caesareans published by the French obstetrician M. Dufeilley. These showed that where the operation was performed in favourable circumstances, 80 per cent of women recovered, compared to only 17 per cent in unfavourable conditions. *The Lancet* commented that these were better results than had been obtained in England, but from 'the semi moribund condition in which the patients generally had been found before the operation' it was surprising that even the small success of 11 per cent maternal survival had been obtained. However, it further concluded that the statistics 'at least prove that the caesarian section need not be the almost certainly mortal operation we were generally thought to consider it'.

At the annual meeting of the British Medical Association (BMA) in

....

83 Young, 1944, p. 142.

1886 there was a discussion of the relative merits of craniotomy and caesarean, and the new Sanger method was not mentioned by the principal speaker. However, W. T. Lusk of New York presented evidence of the improved results with the new technique. In 1887 a death from caesarean was reported at a meeting of the Obstetrical Society of London and the comment was made that, although improved results had been obtained abroad, there had been no comparable improvement in this country (*The Lancet*, 11 June 1887). A liberalisation of attitudes towards the operation occurred in the 1890s. An article based on a meeting appeared in *The Lancet* entitled 'Modern Methods of Caesarean Section' in April 1891. This drew attention to the improvements in the operation brought about by Sanger, whose results were originally published in the United States in 1882 but were not reported in either *The Lancet* or the *British Medical Journal* (*BMJ*). However, his improvement was introduced in 1886 (*The Lancet*, 19 May 1894). The 1891 meeting also disclosed a recent mortality rate of caesarean of 23 per cent. This was above the death rate from craniotomy (at Guy's Hospital this was 16 per cent). So by these statistics craniotomy was still safer; a Dr Herman commented that 'Caesarean section should not replace craniotomy where mortality should not be above normal labour'.

In 1892 a meeting was reported in *The Lancet* where Dr Murdoch Cameron described his experience of performing caesareans. He had carried out fifteen and only two of the women had died; in neither case was their death due to the operation. He described his procedure as follows:

> If labour has not set in it should be induced, then a five or six inch incision in the abdominal wall ought to be made. The uterus is not brought out until the foetus has been extracted. Any rotation is carefully rectified, and a small incision made in the median line until the membranes (which must not be ruptured) are reached. Next the incision is enlarged upwards and downwards, and the child extracted. The uterus is now brought out and thoroughly emptied of placenta and membranes. The edges of the uterine incision are everted by an assistant and deep carbolised silk sutures inserted, with, if necessary a few cat gut ones. (*The Lancet*, 12 March 1892, p. 594)

It was around 1890 that instruments began to be sterilised. Dr Lewers was reported in the *BMJ* in 1911 as saying 'He could remember when in surgical practice generally the instruments were not boiled; this was not much more than 20 years ago, if, indeed, it was quite so long' (4 March).

With this change and the new method of performing the operation, the caesarean section could now be justified more readily, although there was still a great deal of debate about the operation. In 1894 the death rates following the improved techniques of 1886 were given as follows: London – twenty-two caesareans and nine deaths; Glasgow – thirty-two caesareans and five deaths; and the provinces six operations and five deaths (*The Lancet*, 19 May 1894).

Thus the 1870s were a period of great improvement in the operative technique.

CHAPTER THREE

CAESAREANS IN THE TWENTIETH CENTURY

The art and science of midwifery have either been lost
by the younger generation in this country or will
certainly be lost if this mad rage for caesarean section
is continued.

BY the beginning of the twentieth century it was possible to have good results with caesarean section unless women were operated on late in labour, had received repeated vaginal examinations or been subject to other techniques such as failed forceps or external cephalic version. The mortality rate was rapidly diminishing. In Glasgow it was 38 per cent in 1891, 20 per cent in 1902 and 12 per cent in 1904.[1]

A major article appeared in the *Journal of Obstetrics and Gynaecology of the British Empire* in January 1911 by Dr Amand Routh based on a survey of over 100 consultants. It showed the increase in the use of caesareans at Queen Charlotte's Hospital. This had taken two decades, from 1890 to 1909: broadly speaking, these represent the last period before the caesarean was generally performed and the first period when it was adopted more widely. In the last decade of the nineteenth century, out of more than 10,000 deliveries only 7 were carried out by caesarean. In the first decade of this century there were 15,222 deliveries, an increase of 50 per cent, and the numbers of caesareans increased tenfold to 74. The main switch was away from craniotomy, which declined from 28 cases in the first decade to 13 in the second.[2]

The article also drew attention to the way that mortality from the caesarean operation varied according to the condition of the woman. In favourable conditions it was 2.9 per cent, but in suspect ones it was 17.3 per cent. When the woman had previously had a vaginal examination or attempts had been made to deliver by other means, the death rate was 34.3 per cent. The message was that it was better to carry out the operation earlier rather than later, as Radford had suggested almost fifty years previously.[3] Some doctors felt that it was time for caesareans to replace destruction of the

1 Routh, 1911, p. 16.
2 Routh, 1911, p. 17.
3 Routh, 1911, p. 19; Radford, 1865, p. 11.

fetus. In a discussion of the subject in 1911, Hastings Tweedy said it was time that craniotomy on the living child was relegated 'to its place amongst the obsolete barbarities of the past' (*BMJ*, 4 March). However, the maternal mortality rate for high-risk cases of caesarean was such that craniotomy was still safer.

The changes in technique in the early part of the twentieth century meant that there was continuous debate over what the indications for caesarean section should be. R. W. Holmes in 1915 argued that the operation had become a sort of makeshift for real obstetric practice. He pointed out that those who were carrying out caesareans for reasons such as high blood pressure must accept the responsibility for deaths in subsequent pregnancies if the uterus ruptured. He argued that such deaths should be considered in calculating the mortality rates for first caesareans.[4] In 1916 J. T. Williams advocated a caesarean for all cases where there was breech presentation for a primiparous woman, but the same year a cautionary article by F. S. Kellogg entitled 'Caesarean Section Overdone' appeared. Commentators noted that the operation was performed in America for conditions for which British obstetricians would use other methods. In the following year Whitridge Williams told the Clinical Congress of Surgeons of the United States: 'Advances in the practice of medicine and surgery are rarely attained in a thoroughly rational manner, but that a period of undue enthusiasm, or even absurd reckless abuse, usually precedes the establishment of the actual value of a given procedure'.[5]

HOME DELIVERY BY CAESAREAN

On 7 September 1915 a miner's wife had been in labour for fifteen hours with no sign of the head engaging in the pelvis. Her two previous labours had resulted in the sacrifice of the child and Dr Gordon Bell commented thus:

> As the parents were very unwilling to risk the loss of another child, and as the conditions demanded either craniotomy or caesarean section, I elected to do the latter. There was one clean room available; the removal of superfluous ornaments, hangings and furniture was followed by a cleansing with a damp cloth and the spraying of the walls, floor and ceiling with formalin; the room was then closed for two hours; this gave me the nearest approach possible in the circumstances to the surroundings of an operating room. Meantime detailed

4 Young, 1944, p. 164.
5 Young, 1944, pp. 155–7, 165.

preparations were made for the sterilising of all necessary articles. Two drums of sterile dressings and masks can always be at hand but in addition I transported a small Cathcart steriliser which was placed on a gas ring and towels and gowns were steamed, sterilised, and dried in this. Instruments and gloves were easily dealt with in the small portable steriliser contained in most operating bags. The skin of the patient was prepared in the usual way, and after being thoroughly dried was coated with a 2½% solution of iodine in spirit and water.

Preparations were all completed within three hours from the time the message was received, the patient's condition was good, the pains strong and frequent, and re-examination revealed not the slightest progress. The details of the operation scarcely differed from the description in Berkeley and Bonney's 'Gynaecological Operations', and included the use of boiled silk throughout except for skin sutures.

The child, a girl, weighing 8lb was easily removed and breathed at once. It lacked the usual frontal and occipital moulding of the ordinary baby, and therefore looked more like a child a month old. The mother made an uninterrupted recovery; the pulse never rose above 76, and the temperature was normal throughout, not having even the ordinary rise when the milk flow was established on the third day.

I should much have preferred the comfort of a nursing home for this operation, but it was not possible, and I am convinced that many operations involving the transport of the patient by road could quite well be done at home.[6]

STERILISING THE MOTHER AFTER CAESAREAN

Sterilisation after a caesarean was recommended by Blundell in 1819 and he proposed that after the operation the woman should have a portion of her Fallopian tubes removed. In fact in 1830 he suggested that every woman known to have 'contracted pelves' should be sterilised before marriage.[7]

We have seen that the Porro operation entailed the sterilisation of the mother. However, this was common practice even with other kinds of caesarean operation. In 1920 the *BMJ* reported a meeting at which Dr

6 Bell, 1916, pp. 195–6.
7 Routh, 1911, p. 24.

Eardley Holland gave details of 1,089 caesareans which had been followed up. Of these women, 610 had no further pregnancy as 42.6 per cent had been sterilised at the time of the operation. Of the 479 who had a subsequent pregnancy, 91 had not delivered and 42 had had abortions or miscarriages. There had been a total of 396 subsequent births with more than 4 out of 5 of them (82 per cent) being performed by caesarean. Eighteen of the mothers suffered a ruptured scar: this was 3.7 per cent of *all* those with a subsequent pregnancy.[8] It is not clear from his work what percentage of women undergoing a trial of labour suffered a ruptured scar. In fact some confusion arose and in the subsequent debate, Holland's figures were used to support the view that about 4 per cent of women would have a ruptured scar if they attempted a vaginal delivery. This error of interpretation was not pointed out until Chassar Moir wrote to the *BMJ* about it on 9 July 1938.

ONCE A CAESAREAN, ALWAYS A CAESAREAN

The *BMJ* supported this dictum in an editorial in 1922.[9] It argued that there was a very real risk of the rupture of the uterine scar which Eardley Holland's figures put at a 4 per cent risk. The main causes of this were identified as infection of the uterine wound during healing, imperfect methods of suture and improper suture material. Also it drew attention to Professor Munro Kerr's suggestion that with the lower segment operation this risk would diminish as the uterine wall was thinner and could be repaired more easily. However, British obstetricians were reluctant to adopt the new methods and it was not until 1931, when an article by J. St George Wilson of Liverpool was published in which he reported fifty cases with only one death, that their attitudes began to change and the operation came into popular usage.[10] With this development British obstetricians moved away from the policy of repeat caesareans. However, the classical caesarean with the vertical scar still remained important, especially when the emergency was such that the baby had to be extracted quickly. A study of a series of births in nineteen hospitals over the period 1943–47 showed that a classical caesarean was used in over one-fifth (22 per cent) of the operations.[11]

In the United States too, the practice developed of allowing some mothers to have a vaginal birth after a caesarean. In 1944 the *Journal of the American Medical Association* (25 November, p. 855) reported

---

8 Holland, 1920, p. 705.
9 *British Medical Journal*, 1922, p. 278.
10 Young, 1944, p. 217.
11 McIntosh-Marshall, 1949, p. 147.

that out of 496 deliveries of women with a previous caesarean, 109 were delivered vaginally and that these had lengths of labour similar to women approaching their first birth.

DEBATE OVER THE LEVEL OF CAESAREANS

The caesarean operation was becoming safer. Munro Kerr pointed out that, while the maternal mortality rate for women having a caesarean before going into labour was 3.6 per cent in the twenty years up to 1910, it had more than halved to 1.6 per cent in the decade 1911 to 1920.[12] Not surprisingly there was a number of obstetricians arguing for more intervention in childbirth and, in an article entitled 'A Plea for More Frequent Use of Caesarean Section', Dr Arnold Jones spoke of caesareans taking the place of other procedures and of his wish that craniotomy would become 'a relic of a barbaric past'. He continued to suggest that there was no question about the simplicity and safety of the caesarean operation and that the one drawback was the unreliability of the scar in future pregnancies, unless the woman was sterilised (*BMJ*, 16 July 1921).

Inevitably, increased intervention in childbirth led to further concerns over the possible abuse of interventionist techniques. In 1922 the *BMJ* led with a major editorial on caesareans. It commented: 'No subject in obstetrics or gynaecology is being more talked about and discussed at present than caesarean section'.[13] It stated that the increase in popularity was in large part due to the collected statistics of Dr Routh in 1911. It went on to say that there was a danger that the operation could become a panacea for all obstetric ills and quoted a Dr Blacker who said that the ease and safety of the caesarean operation was leading to its abuse.

After considering US evidence, the *BMJ* concluded that there was a temptation to perform an easy, quick and dramatic operation instead of following the safer and better, but more tedious, path of ordinary obstetric methods. It argued that the increased number of indications for the operation, which included varicose veins, abdominal pain and epilepsy, 'is enough to show that the operation is indeed being abused here and now'. It stated the view of one eminent and experienced obstetrician: 'The art and science of midwifery have either been lost by the younger generation in this country or will certainly be lost if this mad rage for caesarean section is continued'.[14]

....

12 Kerr, 1937, p. 523.
13 *British Medical Journal*, 1922, p. 277.
14 *British Medical Journal*, 1922, p. 278.

The *BMJ* conceded that the operation often led to a better outlook for the child, but argued that the profession should not lose its sense of the proportionate value of maternal life as compared to that of the fetus. It said that only in exceptional circumstances was it justified to expose the woman to increased risk in the interests of the unborn child.

The reduced risk of the operation was reflected in a steady decline in operative mortality to 4 per cent by the 1930s. This produced not a decline in the rate of medical intervention in childbirth but rather a move away from the older-style intervention techniques to a surgical procedure that appeared to be proving itself less damaging to the mother and child.

Dame Louise McIlroy said that the operation was much favoured by young surgeons and obstetricians, but commented that giving a trial labour produced valuable information and had reduced the incidence of caesarean in some circumstances, for many women were able to deliver normally.[15]

The changes led to continual debates over the level of operations. One such occurred in 1935 when the British Medical Association had its annual meeting in Melbourne. J. Bright Banister complained that the procedure had degenerated from being a life-saving attempt into an apparently easy way of avoiding difficulties without regard to its perils. There had been an enormous increase in the incidence of the operation, often for such slender reasons as failure to progress, advanced age of the mother, breech and unwillingness to undergo the pains of labour. He argued that from the evidence of 1,763 deliveries in large maternity hospitals in England and 1,723 births in Brooklyn occurring between 1921 and 1926, it appeared that the death rate of the mother for caesarean was 6.6 per cent. For vaginal delivery, it was only 0.45 per cent in England and Wales. He went on to state that in 1932 alone there had been 170 deaths after caesarean.

Dr H. A. Ridler of Sydney agreed that there were too many caesareans: 'This was the result in modern times of the love of the dramatic, of the desire to earn a big fee easily, and of the love of speed.' However, others argued that in using statistics in this way Bright Banister was not comparing like with like, because women having caesarean were often in a very difficult situation anyway. Professor J. B. Dawson said that in Britain there were not too many caesareans, but rather too many done too late. Disasters occurred not after prompt action but after undue delay.[16]

....

15 McIlroy, 1932, p. 796.
16 Bright Banister, 1935, pp. 684–5.

TOO MANY CAESAREANS IN THE UNITED STATES

In 1921 the Massachussets State Medical Society said that caesarean section was the highest cause of maternal death due to puerperal infection.[17] In 1922 the rise in the number of caesareans led to a great deal of opposition. Dr Franklin Newell, Professor of Clinical Obstetrics at Harvard, said that the caesarean was the most abused obstetric operation:

> The operative indication has been a slow though normal labour which the attendant has hastened to end in the manner easiest for himself though often not best for the patient. The increased safety of abdominal surgery, combined with the fact that the operation is much easier to perform than any but the easiest obstetric operation, has caused a loss of perspective and today there is no question but that caesarean section is one of the most abused operations in surgery ... I am convinced that caesarean section as performed by local operators in small communities for the indications furnished by the local practitioner of obstetrics is one of the most fatal of surgical operations.[18]

This represents the first indication that the medical profession was beginning to recognise the possible abuse of the operation in terms of its being used in the interests of the practitioner rather than of the patient.

One very important contribution to the debate was that of Plass, writing in the *American Journal of Obstetrics and Gynecology* in 1931. He stated that, in general, the death rate was 5–10 per cent. In the United States the death rate seems to have been lower, but he estimated a death list each year of 900–1,800, with three-quarters of these being unnecessary.[19]

Two years later, the *BMJ* carried a major article on the subject. It pointed out that in the United States between 1915 and 1929 the neonatal death rate had risen from 3.9 to 5.5 per 1,000 and commented: 'There is little doubt that the great increase in operative deliveries, which has characterised obstetric practice generally during the last 15 years, supplies the explanation for the increased loss of infant life.' It was not just caesareans that had increased but also forceps deliveries, and the *BMJ*'s informant, Professor Plass of Iowa, said that in some hospitals

....

17 Bright Banister, 1935, p. 1143.
18 *British Medical Journal*, 1922, p. 277.
19 Young, 1944, p. 168.

all deliveries were by forceps except 'precipitate delivery' where the baby was born before the obstetrician had a chance to get there (*BMJ*, 13 January, 1934).

In 1933, the New York Academy of Medicine in its report on maternal mortality concluded: 'The data reveal an excessive use of the caesarean section and as a result a great increase in mortality . . . a sharp reduction in the number of caesareans performed is to be recommended.'

In 1934, the White House Conference on Child Health, set up by President Hoover, produced a report which showed that the concerns about unnecessary deaths from caesareans were justified. It showed wide differences in practice. The forceps rate varied between 3.8 per cent in one hospital to 81 per cent in another. The caesarean maternal mortality rate varied a great deal, from 4.2 per cent in Los Angeles to 16.1 per cent in New Orleans. The caesarean mortality rate depended to a large degree on skill of the operator. In one series of just over 100 operations divided equally between obstetricians on the one hand and general practitioners and surgeons on the other, the obstetricians had a maternal mortality rate of 1.8 per cent whereas for the other groups it was 33 per cent. British observers noted that this finding 'illustrates the results which may ensue when men of less skill and experience attempt to follow the example set by obstetricians'. They called for the specialist hospitals to set an example of restraint lest others should try to follow the practice to be 'up to date', with disastrous consequences (*BMJ*, 1934, p. 69).

This theme was maintained in a subsequent article in the *BMJ* which discussed a report on maternal mortality in New York City. It commented: 'The data reveal an excessive use of caesarean section and, as a result, a great increase in mortality.' It recommended a sharp reduction in caesarean section (December 1935).

This reduction did not happen and, during the Second World War, commentators in the United States were still concerned about levels of caesareans. Cotgrove and Norton commented that caesarean section had been frequently used for such reasons as 'primigravidity in the elderly, election by neurotic patients and high social value of the offspring, which can hardly be considered legitimate'.[20] Delee concurred with these sentiments and stated that the high level of operations was a crucial factor in the continuing high maternal mortality rates.[21]

Thus the data in the earlier part of the twentieth century showed great

----

20 Cotgrove and Norton, 1942, p. 201.
21 Delee, 1942, p. 209.

concern among some obstetricians about the caesarean rates which were recognised as being above those necessary for the best care of mothers and their babies; indeed the rates had reached levels where maternal mortality was being increased as a result, rather than being decreased.

CHAPTER FOUR

INTERNATIONAL INFORMATION

One of the major differences between Britain and the United States is that in Britain the midwife still has a strong role and is the senior professional person present in at least three-quarters of births.

THE highest rate of caesareans in the world is in Brazil where nearly one in three (32 per cent) births is by this method. It is followed by Puerto Rico where the rate is three births in ten (29 per cent), with the United States having the third highest level at nearly one birth in four.[1] Some of the information from Brazil is very instructive. In a study of nine hospitals (five in the state of Sao Paulo and four in Rio de Janeiro) it was found that the caesarean rate differs drastically according to payment status: 75 per cent of private patients have caesarean deliveries compared to 42 per cent of insured and 22 per cent of indigent patients.[2] It might be expected that poorer women would have inferior diets and so be more likely to suffer from labour problems. However, private patients were three times as likely to be so classified. In a move to reduce the rate of caesarean delivery the Brazilian government equalised reimbursement fees for both vaginal and abdominal births.[3]

We have been collecting data from different countries and Table 4.1 shows some of the information we have gathered. A striking feature is the great variation between societies of similar social organisation and ethnic types like Sweden and the Netherlands, Czechoslovakia and Hungary, or Scotland and Ireland. Furthermore the Netherlands has consistently had much lower perinatal mortality rates than the United States, despite its low caesarean rate.

In this chapter we consider birth practice in a few selected countries and, as one of the highest rates of caesarean is in the United States, it is with this country that we begin.

....

1 Taffel et al., 1992, p. 22.
2 Janowich, Nakamwa, Entellita, Brown and Clapton, 1982.
3 Carson and Francome, 1983, p. 5.

UNITED STATES   By 1988 the caesarean rate in the United States
————————————   had risen until one in four births were by this
method. This rise has been a subject of public concern, and numerous
publications on the topic have appeared. A US Government Task Force
reported in 1981 that breech presentation, repeat caesarean section and
dystocia were the three diagnoses which had contributed most to the
tripling of the rate between 1968 and 1977 when it was 13.7 per cent.
The Task Force tried to halt the rise.

One of its recommendations was that doctors should end the dictum
'once a caesarean, always a caesarean' and allow a vaginal birth after a
previous caesarean. A second recommendation was for an end to the
increasing trend in the United States of routinely performing a caesarean
for a breech delivery. In 1970 just over one in ten breech births were
performed by caesarean but this increased to six out of ten by 1978.[4]

Table 4.1   *Caesarean rate by year in selected countries 1970–90*

Country	1970	1975	1980	1982	1983	1985	1987	1988	1989	1990
Australia	4.2	8.2	13.2					15.9		
Austria				7.0	7.5					
Belgium				8.0	8.1		9.8			
Canada	5.7	9.6	16.1					19.9		
Czech.	2.3	2.8	4.4	5.2	6.0			8.1		
Denmark	5.7	7.5	10.7	11.7	12.8					
England	4.9			8.2		10.5			12.0	
Fiji			5.2	5.3						
Finland	6.0	8.2						14.4		
France	6.1 (1972)			10.9 (1981)						
Greece									16.7	
Holland	2.1	2.7	4.7	5.3		6.3	6.8	7.2		
Hungary	6.2	6.5		9.2				10.2		
Ireland				6.2						
Israel				10.0 (est.)				10.2		
Italy			11.2		14.5					
Japan		6.4		8.0 (1981)						
New Zealand	3.9			9.8						
Norway	2.2	4.1	7.2	9.0	9.4					
Portugal						11.1	14.1	15.5	16.5	
Scotland		8.1	11.7	12.8				12.8	13.8	14.0
Singapore			14.7							
Spain					11.7 (1986)		12.5	12.3	14.9	
Sweden		7.8	12.0							
USA	5.5	10.4	16.5	18.5	20.3	22.7	24.4	24.7	23.8	23.5
Wales				10.6				12.3	12.4	13.4

....

4 National Institutes of Health, 1982, p. 12.

This was despite the fact that there had been no evidence of a decline in mortality for breech delivery and the report recommended that the vaginal delivery of a breech baby should remain an acceptable choice if the baby is under 8lb in weight and there are no other contraindications.

The committee also recommended studies to promote the accuracy of fetal monitoring and the development of new techniques for making the diagnosis. Furthermore it suggested that the diagnosis of difficult labour should be monitored by peer review.

The report did not succeed in its aim of substantially reducing the number of caesareans. The percentage of women who have a vaginal birth after a caesarean has risen from being only one in twenty-two (4.5 per cent) deliveries after a previous caesarean in 1965. However, the rise, though significant, was only to one in five deliveries of women with a previous caesarean in 1990.[5] Repeat caesarean accounted for over one-third (35.9 per cent) of all caesareans. The proportion of women giving birth by caesarean after a previous one doubled between 1980 and 1988, despite the Task Force's recommendations.

The United States does provide data as to certain age and regional differences in the caesarean rate. The highest rate is in the South where there are six caesareans for every five in the western region. Mothers who are under the age of 20 have just over half the caesarean rate of those over the age of 35. In part this is due to the fact that the younger group will be much less likely to have a repeat caesarean.

One of the important factors is the question of who pays for the operation. If the woman is to pay for the operation herself, the caesarean rate is only one birth in six (16.6 per cent). However, if private insurance is paying, the figure is over one birth in four (25.7 per cent with Blue Cross and 26.1 per cent with other private insurance). Hospitals run for a profit have a caesarean rate of over three births in ten (30.5 per cent), while the state and local government hospitals have a rate of only just over one in five (21.4 per cent). The average stay in hospital for a vaginal delivery was two days, but for a first caesarean it was five days and for a repeat caesarean it was four days.[6]

WHY THE US CAESAREAN RATE IS HIGHER THAN THAT IN BRITAIN

There is evidence from North America that defensive medicine is a major factor underlying the change in mode of delivery. At the time we carried out our

5 Taffel et al., 1992, p. 22.
6 Taffel et al., 1992, p. 22.

survey in Britain, we sent a questionnaire to a number of US doctors and asked them for the reason that the caesarean rate had risen to 24.8 per cent in 1987. Thirty obstetricians responded and all but three (90 per cent) mentioned fear of litigation or made a comment such as 'too many lawyers'. In a detailed letter to us (17 April 1990), Dr Keith Edwards of Bluefield West Virginia wrote in part:

> I am perhaps more familiar with obstetrics in England than some of my colleagues here in America. I stopped doing obstetrics in December 1987. About five years ago I was sued for seven million dollars over a brain-damaged baby. The depositions and other things that occurred in connection with this suit took over two years. Finally we were in a court of law for ten days, and I was completely exonerated by the jury. I continued doing obstetrics and gynaecology for a few years after that, but decided upon reaching the age of fifty-nine that I did not want to do obstetrics any longer.
>
> I think the malpractice risk has caused a lot of people in this country to stop doing obstetrics. Just recently there was a $15 million court judgement against an obstetrician in Charleston, West Virginia. I do not know a great deal about the case but he did a mid-forceps delivery. That obstetrician was carrying a $3 million coverage. It is obvious that this judgement has wiped out all the assets he has acquired in a full lifetime career. Immediately after that I am told that six obstetricians in the city of Charleston closed their obstetric practices and refused to take any new patients, planning to stop doing obstetrics when the ones they had booked had been delivered.
>
> There is no test available which will absolutely tell you whether that child will be in good condition several hours later when that vaginal delivery is accomplished. If the obstetrician decides to wait this out and do a vaginal delivery and he is right, the baby is in good condition: he may get a pat on the back or he may not get any recognition at all. The worst thing that may happen to him is for someone at a Department of Obstetrics and Gynaecology meeting to say that his caesarean section rate is too high. On the other hand, if he miscalculates and follows his patient to delivery and performs a vaginal delivery some three or four hours later and gets a bad baby, he may lose everything that he has ever accumulated in his entire life.

One factor which the US Government Task Force did not stress but which is probably important is the fact that in the United States the vast majority of pregnant women are cared for by obstetricians in private practice.[7]

We have seen that the effect of private practice is to increase intervention rates compared with non-paying patients,[8] and yet the women who can afford to pay for care or insurance are usually taller, less likely to smoke, less likely to be young teenagers, and more affluent. So by all criteria they should be more likely to deliver normally. One important point was noted by Stephenson who drew attention to the fact that in the United States many insurers reimburse doctors by the amount of treatment given.[9] Consequently more tests and procedures per woman mean greater profit.

Differences in physician practice have also been documented in the United States. In a community hospital serving affluent low-risk women which had a 26.9 per cent caesarean rate, it was found that individual physician's rates to range from 19 to 42 per cent without commensurate differences in risk factors or neonatal outcome.[10] In a Wisconsin hospital, with a 14 per cent caesarean rate, individual rates varied from 5.6 to 19.7 per cent with similar lack of correlation between risk factors and outcome.[11] Physician 'style' seemed to be the factor which explained the differences.

In addition, the influence of training and the regionalisation of services into different levels of care have changed the atmosphere in which obstetricians practise. The art of breech delivery, of breech extraction of the second twin following external cephalic version and of mid-forceps delivery is in danger of being lost.[12] One general problem is that doctors usually do not see the effects of their intervention, either in the short term or in the long term, and thus do not always understand the full effect, for example, of performing an episiotomy, let alone a caesarean.

One of the major differences between Britain and the United States is that in Britain the midwife still has a strong role, and is the senior professional present in at least three-quarters of births. A reason that is important in producing a lower caesarean rate here is that it is influenced by the relative status of the birth attendant and the woman giving birth.

7 National Institutes of Health, 1982.
8 DeRegt, Minkoff, Feldman and Schwarz, 1986.
9 Stephenson, 1992, p. 30.
10 Goyert et al., 1989.
11 DeMott and Sandmire, 1990, p. 1593.
12 Olofsson and Rhydstrom, 1985.

If the difference in status between the mother and her carer is large, then the birth attendant's time seems much more important and there will be pressure for a speedy operative delivery. Two doctors writing about the situation in the United States argued that women should not expect doctors to spend too long with them.[13] They were explaining why women should not expect a vaginal birth after a previous caesarean birth (VBAC) and that the related danger meant that the physician must be in constant attendance. This meant: 'Instead of spending the time in the office seeing other patients while you are labouring, the physician must spend many hours exclusively with you, at a time that may be totally inconvenient. Your delivery may take as long as ten hours out of the doctor's day or night while a repeat caesarean would take only an hour or so.' This statement from a practising obstetrician and a gynaecologist shows that there there are clearly other factors than medical ones at work. When midwives are doing the deliveries, their time appears to be less precious and mothers receive treatment based more upon their own needs.

A second difference from the United States is that in Britain there is not just one midwife looking after the woman but a team, so if one person has to go off duty there is another to come and take over. In the United States the woman will usually have just one doctor to look after her care. This can lead to problems when the labour conflicts with other parts of the doctor's life. We will give two examples, one previously published and the other from our own interviews. In the first the woman relates her experience as follows:

> *The nurse said I was 8 cm [dilated] and to begin pushing, so I pushed a little. Then they told me I was completely dilated so I pushed a few times more. The doctor came in then and said I was only 7 cm and not to push. Then they took me to delivery. I assumed it was because it was time to have the baby.*
>
> *Sometime during the day the nurses had told us it was my doctor's birthday and that he was having a party that night. As they were taking me to the delivery room they made my husband wait in the hall. While he was waiting there he heard the doctor say, 'You go ahead without me to the party; I'll be there in 45 minutes.'*
>
> *Then the doctor came into the delivery room and said, 'You might deliver this baby on your own, but it could go on for*

---

13 Hausknecht and Heilman, 1978, p. 35.

a long time and you might still need a C section. The baby's heart tones go down with contractions. It's not real serious but the baby is under a little stress, so it's probably better for the baby that we go ahead and get him out. So I think we should do a C section.' We said OK. Then he gave me the epidural and began the C section. There was no mention of a caesarean to me before that time in the delivery room. I really thought I was going to the delivery room to have a vaginal delivery.[14]

This narrative is similar to what happened at another delivery that occurred on Long Island. At her second delivery the mother, Debbie, waited outside the hospital with her husband in the car until she was within two hours of giving birth because of the poor experience she had had the first time. She went into labour early on a Saturday afternoon and at 1.30 p.m. was 3 cm dilated. The doctor was clearly in a hurry as he had a dinner date at 8.00 p.m. She did not want any drugs but he insisted: 'Otherwise you might be here until tomorrow when I can have this baby in your arms in a few hours.' He also threatened to perform a caesarean section if she did not deliver quickly. Her husband Cliff was upset that his wife's wishes were not being carried out. They told her that they were giving her pitocin (synthetic oxytocin) and put a drip in her arm. Then the labour pains became much greater and she was not able to control them and so needed further drugs as pain-killers. She gave birth to Timothy vaginally at 7.30 p.m. The doctor said it was 'perfect timing' and made a speedy exit. Debbie said, *'I would have liked to have shaken him.'*

These two examples show the effect of having just one caretaker rather than a team. Although in Britain doctors do not usually attend normal deliveries, it does happen on some occasions. Professor Ian Craft was at the Royal Free Hospital and became probably the first person in Britain to deliver a test-tube baby vaginally. He explained in an interview that a crucial factor was 'patience rather than patients' and he related his experience of the previous week: 'I delivered a chief technician after twelve hours at five thirty in the morning. It made me a bit tired during the day. Many would have done a caesarean section at eleven thirty saying "failure to progress".'

There are also training differences between the midwives and doctors which are important. The contrast between the episodic, crisis-orientated

14 Perez, 1989, p. 132.

training of the 1980s US obstetrician and the personal and continuing care of the old-style British domiciliary midwife or GP is striking. The difference in approach resulting from different types of training may be a key factor in different caesarean rates and in reducing the level of unnecessary operations, as it may be possible to recapture the essence of this relationship. Indeed it has not been lost everywhere and the Netherlands is an example of this.[15]

An important difference between Britain and the United States is in the attitudes towards vaginal birth after caesarean (VBAC). In the United States the obstetricians have been and still are much more likely to follow one caesarean by another. Indeed in the United States there was so much resistance to change on this issue that, when a group of obstetricians was asked 'Assuming you could be shown documentation and overwhelming evidence of the safety of permitting labour following caesarean section, would you allow this to alter the management of your patients?', four out of five (80 per cent) answered 'No'. In 1974 in the United States 99 per cent of patients with a previous caesarean had a repeat operation performed. There were attempts to produce change from the professional hierarchy. In 1982 the American College of Obstetricians and Gynecologists (ACOG) called for VBACs to occur in hospitals which had the following characteristics: they were to be capable of caring for high-risk mothers; to have 24-hour blood banking; electronic fetal monitoring; on-site anaesthesia coverage; and the continuous presence of a surgeon.

Some obstetricians also reported moving away from the established position in that year. Thus Porrecco said that it was from this time that, at his hospital in Denver, he stopped offering elective repeat caesareans to women who were candidates for labour. He commented: 'in my view there is little difference between offering elective repeat caesarean sections and offering elective primary caesarean sections to women who wish to avoid labor'.[16]

Two years later the ACOG conditions had been reduced to electronic fetal monitoring and the general requirement to respond to obstetric emergencies. In 1988 the percentage of VBACs had increased to 12.6 per cent. That year the ACOG published new guidelines for their performance. This dropped any mention of fetal monitoring and argued that a woman with one previous caesarean delivery with a low transverse incision should be encouraged to attempt labour in her second pregnancy. Furthermore, those with two previous caesareans who wished to try for a vaginal birth should not be discouraged. It also specified that a previous classical uterine

....
15 Young, 1987.
16 Porrecco, 1990, p. 151.

incision should be a contraindication to labour and that the hospital should be capable of performing a caesarean within thirty minutes, should one become necessary.[17] Due in part to these guidelines, in 1989 there was a large jump in the VBAC rate to 18.5 per cent. There was a smaller increase in 1990 but this brought the rate to over one in five births (20.4 per cent) for the first time ever.[18] Individual hospitals have shown a much greater change in some cases. For example, the University Medical Center of Jacksonville (Florida) had a fall in its overall caesarean rate from 28 per cent of deliveries to 11 per cent between 1986 and 1989. In part this was because its overall VBAC rate increased from 21 to 70 per cent of deliveries after previous caesarean.[19]

In 1988 E. Philipp said that it was still a majority of US obstetricians who followed a policy of 'once a caesarean, always a caesarean'. Interestingly, when we wrote to 150 US obstetricians and received replies from 30 who were still practising, only one said he supported 'once a caesarean, always a caesarean' and 27 said they did not agree with it, with 2 leaving this question blank. It could be that those who responded were more inclined towards conservative obstetric practice. However, it is more likely that at last doctors have realised that this dictum is untenable in the face of the evidence from the research and the recommendations of the ACOG.

It must be said that, although obstetricians are now not nominally following this dictum in the United States, they are still being very restrictive in their support of a VBAC for the individual woman. In fact Shearer proposes that, like all labouring women, VBAC mothers require close careful attention during active labour. However, she suggests: 'Perhaps what should be required is not electronic fetal monitoring but midwifery care'.[20]

So we have seen a variety of reasons for the higher caesarean rate in the United States. One final point is that in the United States many people believed by the late 1970s that a growth in caesareans was progressive. Dr Pennington of Nassau County, Long Island, told us of the divisions and conflicts as he opposed some of the more active of his colleagues. A statement which received publicity in the United States actually emanated from a British journal but the fashion for which it called became much more prevalent in America:

Planned delivery, elective induction, and acceleration of labour are not simply progress in purely medical terms, but also

....
17 American College of Obstetricians and Gynecologists, 1988; Shearer, 1992, p. 34.
18 Taffel et al., 1992, p. 22.
19 Sanchez-Ramos, Kaunitz, Peterson, Martinez-Schnell and Thompson, 1990, p. 1081.
20 Shearer, 1992, p. 34.

socially acceptable to both mother and obstetrician. It is more satisfactory to the mother if she knows exactly when she is to have her baby, how long she is likely to be in hospital, when she needs to ask for relatives' help in caring for her present family and when her husband needs holiday time off work. Taking this argument further, not only will elective induction of labour for purely social reasons become more readily available, but elective delivery by caesarean section might at some later date be contemplated for the same reasons.[21]

This attitude has not become widespread but in the places where this approach has been accepted, there have been much higher caesarean rates as we have seen in parts of the United States and in Brazil.

CANADA   In Canada the caesarean rate rose from one in eighteen
————————   deliveries (5.7 per cent) in 1970 to one in five in 1988 (19.9 per cent). Health care is funded by a government insurance scheme with universal coverage for all aspects of care. Childbirth takes place almost completely in hospital with less than 1 per cent of deliveries occurring at home and a small number in birth centres.[22] Because the population of Canada is concentrated in the large urban centres near the US border, it is often necessary for women from the rest of the country to travel long distances to give birth. This is especially problematical because Canada was for some time the only country in the world without a legalised system of midwifery care.

In 1986 the Canadians published a statement following a national consensus conference on aspects of caesarean birth which was circulated widely in an attempt to reduce the national caesarean rate. They set criteria for vaginal breech delivery, for VBAC and the diagnosis of difficult labour, as well as defining areas which required further research. A year later little change had occurred and more direct action was being piloted in an attempt to influence doctors to change their practice.[23] This educational exercise also failed but a later initiative, using a peer group leader, has been successful in reducing the rate of caesareans.[24]

One of the reasons for the rise in the caesarean rates may well have been the decline in the number of deliveries carried out by family phys-

....

21 Sutherst and Case, 1975, p. 241.
22 Enkin, 1991.
23 Lomas, 1988.
24 Lomas, 1991.

icians. By 1990 they were performing less than a third of deliveries and the trend was towards specialist obstetrician/gynaecologists. Family doctors give a number of reasons for stopping obstetric practice. One is the conflict with family life of having to carry out deliveries in unsocial hours and a second is the high malpractice insurance that has to be paid by family doctors who practise obstetrics.[25] This has led to a serious shortage of medical providers of obstetric care.

Another reason for the high rate of caesareans in Canada is that, although things may be beginning to change, it largely follows the practice of 'once a caesarean, always a caesarean' which obtained in the United States. In fact, only one community hospital in nine will allow a woman to try for a vaginal birth after a caesarean. In regional hospitals practice is more liberal and almost half (46 per cent) will allow a woman to try for a normal delivery.

The shortage of doctors and the changes in attitudes towards delivery have led to a strong demand for midwifery care. Midwifery existed in the early days in Canada but had almost disappeared by the end of the nineteenth century because of medical opposition and legislation. One suggestion was that doctors began incorporating midwifery within their practices after seeing how lucrative it could be. They succeeded in convincing pregnant women that childbirth needed medical assistance and midwives began to be regarded as unsafe practitioners. As women were denied access to medical schools, only men were trained as doctors and so childbirth was taken over by men in a way which also happened, but to a lesser degree, in the United States. The revival of midwifery owes its roots to the counter-culture movement of the 1960s as women began to seek a more natural state in life and began to question the high level of technical intervention in childbirth.[26] Although not legalised it has become increasingly well organised since the mid-1970s.[27] In 1986 the Ontario government announced its intention of licensing midwifery as an autonomous, self-governing profession. One estimate is that by the mid-1990s around one woman in twenty in Ontario would be delivered by a midwife and the implication is that this figure would increase.[28] The movement towards midwifery care should help reduce the number of unnecessary caesareans in Canada.

....

25 Enkin, 1991, p. 16.
26 Solderstrom, Chamberlain, Kaitell and Stewart, 1990.
27 Enkin, 1991, p. 17.
28 Kaufmann, 1990, p. 144.

AUSTRALIA   The best estimates indicate that the percentage of deliveries by caesarean rose from 4.2 per cent in 1970 to 16.9 per cent in 1986 and so increased four times over the period. However, in part these figures are estimates as there are no uniform sources of data providing national figures for caesarean rates. The 1986 figure is the first national study of caesarean section rates, made possible by combining 1986 data from hospital morbidity collections and Medicare claims. Tasmania could not be included. The date also showed that there were wide variations in the rates between hospitals. Rates were generally higher in the capital cities and for women who had insurance.[29] The highest rates were in Canberra (26.3 per cent) and Brisbane (25.4 per cent). The rates for Northern Territory, South Australia and Queensland were higher than the rates for other states.

An article on Western Australia showed that over the seven-year period 1980–87, emergency sections increased from 5.9 per cent of all deliveries to 8.2 per cent but that elective sections had a larger percentage rise from 5.3 to 8.7 per cent. This gives a total caesarean rate of 16.9 per cent which is above the estimates for Australia as a whole.[30] However, despite the trend to more intervention there was indication that more women wanted home births. The percentage of planned home births rose from 3.5 per 1,000 deliveries in 1981 to 8.0 in 1987. Although these women who planned home births were similar in their number of previous children and marital status and were in fact older, their caesarean rate was much lower than average at 4.2 per cent.[31] From this evidence it seems likely that any further movement towards home deliveries could reduce the caesarean rates.

IRELAND   In Ireland home birth is unusual but the tradition of midwifery stemming from the eighteenth century, when obstetricians wrote textbooks of midwifery, is still strong and visitors to the National Maternity Hospital are struck by the quiet, uncluttered labour ward and the respect for the midwives. In an interesting article Boylan drew attention to the fact that in 1968 Kieran O'Driscoll was elected Master at the National Maternity Hospital.[32] The Master is a senior consultant who has control of the hospital for a seven-year period during which time he or she can set policies in all areas of the hospital. O'Driscoll had a particular interest in preventing long labour because he was

29   Renwick, 1991, p. 300.
30   Read, Waddell, Prendiville and Stanley, 1991.
31   Woodcock, Read, Moore, Stanley and Bower, 1991, p. 31.
32   Boylan, 1989.

worried about the plight of women who were in labour for over thirty-six hours, became dehydrated and confused and often experienced a traumatic delivery after a long period of time. He aimed to reduce the level of stress by bringing down the time for labour and over the years the definition of prolonged labour was reduced to twelve hours. However, no strict time limit was placed on labour and if a woman had not delivered during that period, she did not automatically undergo a caesarean – she was just regarded as being in prolonged labour.[33]

In the Dublin Maternity there is a commitment to low levels of intervention among all the staff members. The midwives are in charge of the day-to-day running of the hospital and junior doctors are there to learn from them. Boylan comments:

> *The junior physicians are regarded as postgraduate students, whose function is to learn, not to teach; they do not know enough to teach. I trained in that system, and found it very reassuring to go onto a labour ward floor knowing very little about the supervision of labour, but meeting one of the head nurses who did know all about it and learning from her.*[34]

The active approach to labour in Dublin included breaking the waters to assess their quality and colour. If clear, they assume that fetal distress is unlikely, but if stained with the baby's faeces (meconium) then the woman is regarded as being in a different category and in need of greater supervision and monitoring.

The Dublin evidence on caesareans is instructive. O'Driscoll and Foley reported that, during the years 1965–80 when caesarean rates increased dramatically in centres across the United States from less than 5 per cent to more than 15 per cent,[35] the Dublin caesarean rate rose only from 4.2 to 4.8 per cent and perinatal mortality rate (PMR) fell from 42.1 to 16.8 per 1,000 for infants born weighing 500 g or more, which is a greater fall than occurred in the United States. They concluded that these results did not support the contention that the increase in caesarean births had contributed significantly to the decline in perinatal mortality.

When the Dublin approach to labour was introduced in Houston, Texas, the duration of labour was reduced from an average of nearly thirteen hours to nearly eight and the caesarean rate fell from over one birth in five (23 per cent) to one birth in ten (10 per cent).

....

33 Boylan, 1989, p. 114.
34 Boylan, 1989, p. 115.
35 O'Driscoll and Foley, 1983.

CZECHOSLOVAKIA   Stembera looked at caesarean rates and the
───────────────────   PMR in mature babies in the various provinces
in Czechoslovakia in 1986.[36] Overall the caesarean rate was 6.5 per cent,
with variation between 4 and 7 per cent. The PMR of normally formed
babies over 3,000 g was found to fall from 1.5 to 1.0 per 1,000 births
as the caesarean rate rose from 4 to 7 per cent.

In a later article Stembera noted a caesarean rate of 7.8 per cent in
the Czech Republic which is less than a third of the US rate, and the
perinatal mortality rates are not increased by the low rates.[37] In fact the
author maintains that in many instances caesarean section can put at
risk the mother and the neonate. The main indications for caesarean
were the hazard of fetal hypoxia and unfavourable presentation of the
fetus.

HOLLAND   Treffers and Laan showed no relationship between place
─────────   of delivery and PMR in the different regions of Holland
between 1980 and 1983.[38] The caesarean rate was not given but the rate
of home confinement ranged from 24.3 to 50.8 per cent and the PMR
from 10.5 to 12.1 per 1,000. This also suggests indirectly that beyond a
certain minimum level of caesareans the PMR would not decline further.

After birth the midwife is assisted by a maternity aide who helps
with shopping and children as well as checking the woman's physical
condition.[39] This enables the midwife to perform eighty or more births
per year and to provide a very personal service to a woman she knows
and stays with throughout labour. Most of the hospitals are small.[40]

CHILDBIRTH IN THE LESS   Women in the poorer countries have
DEVELOPED WORLD   much larger family sizes on average. In
─────────────────────   1987 the average woman had over six
children in Iran, Zimbabwe, Pakistan, Nigeria and Ethiopia. The average
size was over seven children in Zambia, Tanzania, Jordan and Afghani-
stan. In Kenya the average woman had eight children. Data from the
world fertility survey showed that many of these births were due to lack
of access to family planning and that if every woman who wanted to
use birth control could get it, the birth rate in the poor countries would

....

36 Stembera, 1987.
37 Stembera, 1992.
38 Treffers and Laan, 1986.
39 Van Teijlingen, 1990.
40 Phaff, 1986.

reduce by more than a third.[41] The poorer level of general health and care and the high number of babies, very often without spacing between births to give the woman time to recover, are factors which lead to many more maternal deaths. In 1991 the British government published data suggesting that the number of maternal deaths per 1,000 births were 6.4 in Africa, 4.2 in Asia and 2.7 in Latin America, compared with a current rate of 0.07 in the United Kingdom.[42] These data suggest that the average birth is ninety times as dangerous in Africa and sixty times as dangerous in Asia as it is here. This kind of evidence shows the great amount that needs to be done world-wide to improve maternal health.

In Nigeria analysis of data of 1,500 pregnant women who went to a teaching hospital without being booked for antenatal care revealed four main categories of care providers. These are traditional birth attendants, trained midwives in maternity centres, medical officers in state hospitals and obstetricians working in conjunction with other paramedical workers in tertiary centres.[43]

A study of Jos University Teaching Hospital showed a caesarean rate of 4.4 per cent over two years of study. This was a relatively low rate but unfortunately there was a very high PMR of 235 per 1,000 births. The obstetricians are trying to implement changes to reduce this.[44] There has been a policy of training the traditional birth attendants to help improve their practices, the standardisation of referral procedures and seminars for all those working in the primary obstetric health care system. Preliminary results show an encouraging sign of reduction in perinatal mortality.

An important article on general antenatal care in developing countries looked at the prevention of neonatal tetanus which the authors rightly argued should be a strong objective of prenatal care – all women should be immunised against tetanus.[45] After studying the information from twenty-four developing countries they found that, of women attending for prenatal care, 72 per cent were immunised in a sample of fourteen African countries, 85 per cent in two Asian countries and 47 per cent in eight Latin American and Caribbean countries. There is clearly scope for improving care and protecting women and their babies.

....

41 Francome, 1990a, p. 9.
42 Department of Health, 1991.
43 Omu, 1991, p. 70.
44 Wright, Kapu and Onwuhafua, 1991.
45 Beukins, Tsui, Kotelchuck and Degraft-Jonson, 1991, p. 121.

CHAPTER FIVE

WHY A CAESAREAN MAY BE NECESSARY

. . . the evidence suggests that once a caesarean rate has risen to about 6–8 per cent any further increase does not improve the health of either mothers or babies

WE have seen that the caesarean rate varies a great deal between different countries, hospitals and individual obstetricians. Thus some women will have the operation, often before labour begins (elective caesarean) while other women presenting with identical or similar problems in another setting will be encouraged to deliver vaginally and often do so. To account for these differences we can divide the reasons for performing a caesarean into two separate categories – the absolute reasons for which women will always need a caesarean and the relative indications where practice will vary.

ABSOLUTE REASONS FOR A CAESAREAN

The majority of women will have a normal labour and be able to give birth vaginally. However, there are situations where the only safe option for either the mother or the baby, or for both, is to have a caesarean.

Insufficient room for the baby (feto-pelvic disproportion)

Historically, the condition most often occurring is that where the baby's head is too large to pass through the pelvic bones. This may be due to the size or position of the baby or the size or shape of the mother's pelvis. Women under 5 feet tall tend to have a smaller pelvis, although some of them also have smaller babies. In other cases, the pelvis may be an abnormal shape: if, for example, the mother has previously fractured her pelvis or had rickets as a child. This condition is much less common than it was. As can be seen from Chapter 2, in the eighteenth and nineteenth centuries poorer nutrition meant that rickets often caused pelvic deformity.

Where feto-pelvic disproportion is suspected, it has been common practice to assess the relative sizes of the outlet of the pelvis and the baby using clinical palpation, X-rays and/or ultrasound. Unfortunately, recent studies have shown increasingly that such attempts to assess whether or not the baby can pass through the pelvis are unreliable predictors since some women whose pelves have been shown to be 'radiologically inadequate' have succeeded in giving birth vaginally, and some women whose pelves have been shown to be 'radiologically adequate' have required emergency caesareans.[1] Another factor has been that even where a woman's pelvis is assessed to be adequate for vaginal delivery, her obstetrician may nevertheless advise her to have an elective caesarean. Thus, unless the woman's pelvis is clearly shown to be inadequate, the balance of evidence is currently in favour of encouraging the woman to deliver vaginally.

Another condition for which a caesarean is necessary is for a transverse lie with shoulder presentation (see illustration on page 62). Some doctors are beginning to attempt to turn such babies to a more favourable position for vaginal delivery using external cephalic version before labour. However, this practice requires further evaluation.[2]

As discussed in Chapter 3, some US doctors used to perform a caesarean whenever the baby was in the breech position (see illustration on page 62) but this has become less common since a government report attacked the practice.[3] They were thus treating a breech position as an absolute indication for performing a caesarean and, as we shall see in Chapter 8, this attitude is still taken by some British obstetricians. In fact, breech position is one of the relative indications for a caesarean and we therefore discuss it in more detail on page 70.

Other absolute reasons for performing a caesarean are where access to the pelvis is blocked by fibroids or an ovarian cyst.

Problems with the baby

There are times when the baby is threatened and a caesarean is necessary. If, for example, the placenta is situated in the lower part of the uterus (placenta praevia) or if there is bleeding behind the placenta which then separates from the uterus wall (abruptio placenta), a caesarean may be necessary and sometimes the decision is taken as a matter of urgency.

Midwives and doctors keep a check on the baby's well-being during pregnancy. If poor growth is noted then this can be checked by an ultrasound scan – the method of using high-frequency sound waves to produce a picture

....

1 Krishnamurthy, Fairlie, Cameron, Walker and MacKenzie, 1991.
2 Hofmeyr, 1991.
3 National Institutes of Health, 1982.

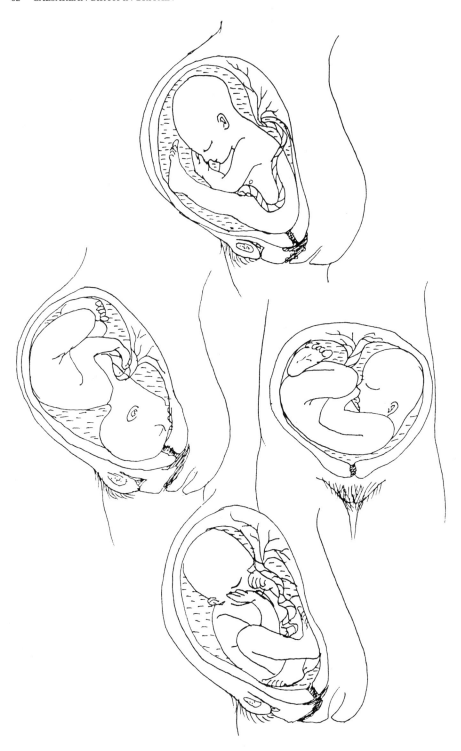

of the baby. The mother herself may also suspect something is wrong if the baby becomes less active. Although all babies have periods of activity and inactivity, several days of reduced or no activity can be important. The condition of the baby can be assessed by measuring its heart rate using an electronic fetal monitor. This is used to print out a chart or 'trace' showing not only the baby's heart rate, but also the response of the baby to uterine contractions and other stimuli ('variability'). More specialised Doppler ultrasound scanning equipment can be used to measure the blood flow between the baby and the placenta which is responsible for conveying both oxygen and food to the baby. Where small babies are due to intra-uterine growth retardation, doctors must distinguish between small normal babies that can be allowed to deliver vaginally and those who have used up all their reserves of fuel and need to be delivered by caesarean.

If the baby shows signs of fetal distress during labour, such as abnormalities in the heart rate or the passing of fresh meconium, further evidence of how much oxygen the baby is getting can be obtained from a fetal blood sample taken from the baby's head. Fetal blood sampling can be performed only when the waters have broken spontaneously or have been artificially ruptured. Research shows that in labour, doubtful fetal heart rates should always be checked by fetal blood sampling,[4] but unfortunately not every maternity unit or practitioner follows this policy. In addition, although the use of electronic fetal monitoring is almost universal in British maternity units, 55 per cent of units lacked fetal blood sampling equipment in 1992.[5]

Problems with the placenta

If the placenta is lying low in the uterus it is called 'placenta praevia' and may block the passage of the baby and cause heavy bleeding. In fact the first sign of placenta praevia is bleeding from the vagina which can occur without any pain in the abdomen. The position of the placenta is confirmed by ultrasound and an elective caesarean will be needed either when the baby is mature at about thirty-eight weeks or earlier as an emergency if the bleeding is too heavy. If the diagnosis is made by ultrasound scan alone, a vaginal examination can be performed in the labour ward theatre without anaesthesia, but with everything prepared for a caesarean. This will confirm whether there is a placenta praevia and whether this is completely covering the cervix. If not, the waters can be broken and the woman can be allowed to labour naturally.

....
4 Chalmers et al., 1989.
5 Balen and Smith, 1992.

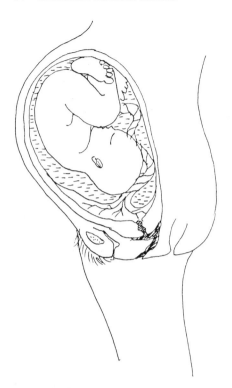

A second problem with the placenta which can occur is when part of it peels away from the uterus causing sudden pain in the abdomen and bleeding from the vagina. This is called placental abruption and is more likely to occur in a woman who has high blood pressure. If there is only a small amount of bleeding, the condition often rights itself and the pregnancy can be allowed to continue with careful checking to ensure that the placenta is transferring enough oxygen to the baby. If the bleeding is heavy, the baby may need to be rescued urgently by an emergency caesarean.

It is therefore important for the woman to see a doctor straight away if there is any bleeding from the vagina during pregnancy.

Problems with the mother's health

Since the Second World War, the proportion of caesareans performed for fetal indications has increased. However, it nevertheless remains the case that some maternal diseases can require a caesarean. High blood pressure can exist before, but more often develops during pregnancy. If it should occur, it normally develops after twenty-four weeks, and especially between twenty-eight and thirty-four weeks, and gets better after birth. If the blood pressure becomes excessively high it is called pre-eclampsia (or 'pre-eclamptic toxaemia') and may be associated with excessive weight gain (more than 26 lb over the pregnancy), swelling of the ankles and fingers (oedema) and protein in the urine. This is why all antenatal checks include measuring the blood pressure, testing the urine and feeling the woman's hands and feet for swelling. If the blood pressure rises too high it can effect the functioning of the placenta and slow down the baby's growth or cause the placenta to separate from the uterus, causing sudden pain in the abdomen and bleeding from the vagina. It can also harm the mother, causing fits (eclampsia). An alternative explanation of pre-eclampsia is that poor formation of the placenta early in pregnancy causes raised blood pressure as the woman's body over-compensates for its poor functioning.[6]

If the mother has previously suffered a stroke or has a particular physical disability, an increase in blood pressure from pushing out the baby in the second stage of labour could be dangerous. Occasionally other medical conditions such as heart disease or diabetes may give rise to problems during pregnancy, leading doctors to advice a caesarean.

How often is a caesarean absolutely indicated?

The proportion of deliveries that require to be delivered by caesarean is based on 1980s data from a variety of sources including Ferguson and data from the Royal London Hospital.[7] Adding together the indications described above makes a total primary caesarean rate of between 5.8 and 8.5 per cent for singleton births. Francome and Huntingford, writing in 1980, concluded that 'it should be a cause for concern if rates rise above 6% of births'. This figure now seems very low in comparison with current practice, although the evidence suggests that once a caesarean rate has risen to about 6–8 per cent any further increase does not improve the health of either mothers or babies. Midwifery evidence also suggests that the obstetric view of what is a reasonable rate may be too high.[8]

Birth trauma as a cause of death had fallen from 8.9 per cent of all perinatal deaths in 1958 (a rate of 3.0 per 1,000) to 1.1 per cent in 1970 (a rate of 0.4 per 1,000), during which time the caesarean rate almost doubled, rising from 2.7 to 4.5 per cent,[9] and the PMR fell from 33 to 23 per 1,000. Thus birth trauma as a cause of death around the time of birth had virtually been eliminated by 1970 and the further rises in the caesarean rate since this time have probably had little effect in lowering the perinatal deaths for this reason.

RELATIVE INDICATIONS FOR A CAESAREAN

Relative indications for a caesarean are the more loosely defined conditions of fetal distress and 'failure to progress' or dystocia (difficult labour), which seem to have been diagnosed with increasing frequency over the last thirty years. These two indications were responsible for almost half of the rise in the US caesarean rate from

....

6 Redman and Walker, 1992.
7 Ferguson, 1985.
8 Durrand, 1992.
9 Butler and Bonham, 1963; Chamberlain and Chamberlain 1975.

5.5 per cent in 1970 to 15.7 per cent in 1978. Thirty per cent of the rise was due to fetal distress being diagnosed and 10–15 per cent to 'dystocia'.[10] It could be argued that the increasing medicalisation of childbirth and the fragmentation of care, which often mean that women labour in an alien environment, cared for by a large team of health professionals they do not know, have created conditions in which women find it more difficult to labour efficiently.

Fetal distress   Fetal distress is the condition where the baby in the uterus, for a variety of reasons, is not receiving enough oxygen. The causes of fetal distress include a placenta not supplying enough oxygen to the baby; unnaturally strong contractions of the uterus which may result from the use of synthetic oxytocin; and compression of the umbilical cord. Fetal distress can occur either before or during labour. If the condition becomes acute, the baby may have brain damage from lack of oxygen or may die. Fetal distress usually manifests itself in abnormalities in the fetal heart rate. These can be picked up by measuring the baby's heartbeat using a fetal stethoscope, Sonicaid or electronic fetal monitor. Variability of the heart rate which is also usually affected in fetal distress can be assessed by looking at the trace from an electronic fetal monitor. Before labour, Doppler ultrasound scanning equipment can be used to measure the blood flow which supplies oxygen to the baby; during labour, a sample of blood may be taken from the baby's scalp to check the acid level in the baby's blood which indicates more accurately whether the baby is short of oxygen. The passing of fresh meconium can also indicate fetal distress, although this is not always the case.

Despite the growth in the use of electronic fetal monitoring in the last twenty years, it is still difficult to diagnose whether a baby is in distress because the evidence from electronic fetal monitoring can be difficult to interpret. As we have seen, fetal blood sampling can be used to help reduce the number of false alarms and unnecessary caesareans, but some maternity units do not have fetal blood sampling equipment or do not use it frequently enough.

Acute fetal distress in labour occurs in about one birth in 100 in hospital practice.[11] In another study of eighty-four independent birth centres it was found that in a series of 11,814 deliveries between 1985 and 1987, one in fifty-six women (1.8 per cent) had babies with sustained

....

10 National Institutes of Health, 1982, p. 7.
11 Zuspan, Quilligan, Iams and van Geijn, 1979.

fetal distress. In this study the overall caesarean rate was 4.4 per cent and fetal distress was the reason for 16.5 per cent of these operations. In the United States as a whole, different studies have shown that between one in four and one in eight caesareans were due to fetal distress (12–24 per cent), often diagnosed using electronic fetal monitoring alone.

What is dystocia (or difficult labour) and how long is long?

Medical ideas of what constitutes a long labour vary. In the British Birth Survey of 1958, twenty-four hours was considered long but by 1970, eighteen hours was taken as the time beyond which a labour was deemed long.[12] At the National Maternity Hospital in Dublin, doctors have followed a policy of intervening energetically by rupturing the membranes and giving syntocinon where labour promises to last longer than twelve hours. This policy is known as the 'active management of labour' and has influenced the practice of many British obstetricians and hospitals.

As is shown in Chapter 8, almost nine in ten of the British obstetricians replying to our survey said they did not have 'a time-limit in labour after which a caesarean is normally performed'. Of the thirty-nine who did have a time limit, just over half (twenty) said they had a limit of twelve hours. One British consultant said he considered the labour long and the woman in need of a caesarean 'if the sun had set twice on her labour'. The longest time mentioned was by one consultant who set a time limit of thirty-six hours.

The National Maternity Hospital in Dublin pioneered the active management of labour, keeping labour shorter than twelve hours and yet kept the caesarean rate below 7 per cent. Although different forms of so-called active management are used freely in the United Kingdom, our study shows that few obstetricians have adopted this time limit and yet the caesarean rate is almost twice that in Dublin. Anecdotal evidence suggests that where active management in UK hospitals conforms more closely to the Dublin approach, caesarean rates are lower, at around 10 per cent.

One factor which is often overlooked when deciding clinically whether a labour is long, is the accurate diagnosis of the onset of established or 'active' labour after the early or 'latent' phase of labour. In Dublin, the twelve hours permitted for labour do not begin to run until the woman is diagnosed as being in active labour. Active labour is not deemed to begin until the cervix is 3 cm dilated and fully 'effaced' or flattened, and

....

12 Butler and Bonham, 1963; Chamberlain and Chamberlain, 1975.

the woman is having strong, regular contractions. Before that time, the woman may be encouraged to return home until the contractions become stronger. Once a woman is in the active phase of labour, she has one midwife allocated to her who gives her positive support and encouragement. This midwife is able to stay with the woman until the birth because labour will not be allowed to last longer than twelve hours. It is possible that this active support may itself affect the duration of labour. Randomised controlled trials showed that women who were allocated a birth companion needed less oxytocin and fewer epidurals and caesarean sections.[13]

Where some UK hospitals may be falling down in their application of the true active management of labour is in a less strict diagnosis of the onset of the active phase. Even in hospitals where there is not an explicit policy of active management, it is common for timing of the length of labour to begin before the end of the latent phase. Thus it is more likely for a labour to be perceived as being 'long' and for unnecessary intervention to occur, culminating in an increased caesarean rate: the 'cascade of intervention'.[14]

Another factor which may account for the low caesarean rate in Dublin is that inductions are not performed unless the condition of the woman's cervix is favourable for labour. We are not advocating that every maternity unit should have a policy of active management based on that at Dublin, but rather we suggest that there may be other factors in the care of women which may be keeping the caesarean section rate low.

The evidence does not suggest that fairly long labours have a detrimental affect on babies. In the British Birth Survey of 1958, the PMR did not rise until labour had lasted over twenty-four hours in a multigravid woman and over forty-eight hours in a primigravida. These are only one in twenty-five (4 per cent) and one in thirty-seven (2.7 per cent) respectively of each group in the population. We would not advocate labours lasting as long as two days, but there are now ways of helping women to deliver earlier. In 1970 in England and Wales labour was longer than twenty-four hours in only one birth in twenty (5.1 per cent). This might be thought surprising, as only 0.6 per cent of labours were accelerated using oxytocin. In today's conditions some of these longer dysfunctional labours would be shortened by augmentation with oxytocin and many of the rest would be associated with feto-pelvic disproportion.

....

13 Kennell, Klaus, McGrath, Robertson and Hinckley, 1991, p. 2197.
14 Inch, 1989.

Multiple births   Twins account for about one in eighty births in the
─────────────   United Kingdom and the incidence of triplets is normally about one in 6,000. It is usually safe for twins and triplets to be
born vaginally although triplets are usually born by caesarean today.
Quadruplets and higher-order births are usually born by caesarean, but
the evidence for this practice is scant. Concern has been expressed about
the increase in grand multiple births owing to the wider use of assisted
conception.[15] The caesarean rate has risen for twins, in particular the
second twin, but this rise does not seem justified by the evidence.[16]

With multiple pregnancies the mother may be very uncomfortable
because of the size of the uterus. She also tends to be tired and anaemic
as the developing babies use up her reserves of iron and vitamins. This
can be counteracted by the woman paying careful attention to her diet
and by taking extra iron and vitamins during pregnancy. There is an
increased tendency to develop high blood pressure and the mother may
go into labour prematurely if the uterus is overstretched. There is also
more chance that one of the babies will be breech or even lie sideways
in the uterus (transverse lie). From a statistical point of view, it seems
unlikely that there would be a significant contribution to the overall
caesarean rate from twin pregnancies. Even if the rate were to be doubled
from 10 to 20 per cent, this would only increase the overall rate by 0.1
per cent.

Smaller and larger babies   Smaller babies are much more likely to die
─────────────────   than larger ones. While only one in fifteen
babies are under 2.5 kg, almost three in five (60 per cent) of the deaths
are to such small babies.[17] Many of the very low birthweight babies will
be delivered by caesarean because of malpresentation, fetal distress,
heavy bleeding before birth ('antepartum haemorrhage') or pre-
eclampsia, and it is unlikely that this group would contribute significantly
to the overall caesarean rate. In the Scottish survey, 2.2 per cent of
caesareans were performed on babies before thirty-two weeks.[18] Another
group of infants now included in this category are those born before
twenty-eight weeks. In our 1990 survey, only one in twenty-eight obstetricians said they would normally carry out a caesarean at twenty-four
weeks for fetal distress and another one in five said it depends on the

....

15 Levene, 1986.
16 Rydhstrom, Ingemarsson and Ohrlander, 1990.
17 Office of Population Censuses and Surveys, 1990.
18 McIlwaine et al., 1985.

circumstances. At twenty-six weeks, however, nearly one in three answered 'yes', and only one in seven said they would not carry one out. These practices seem to us to show a reasonable assessment of the chance of intact survival of the baby with increasing gestation. A number of recent studies have looked critically at the delivery of premature babies by caesarean and begun to assess other ways of managing a very premature delivery. Where the membranes are intact and the amniotic fluid is able to protect the premature baby's soft head from the pressures of labour, vaginal delivery may be a safer alternative than delivery through a rigid uterine scar.

Sometimes there may be disproportion if the baby is very large, and sometimes a woman who has had several babies, with each one growing larger, may reach a size where she cannot deliver. Despite more sophisticated ultrasound scanning equipment, it is still difficult to estimate a baby's size and weight accurately. Fortunately, the problem of large babies does not appear to be increasing. In the Third World, the grand-multiparous woman (who has had more than four babies), whose uterus is thinned by repeated childbearing, often ruptures the uterus and both mother and baby die.

Breech babies As mentioned above, some obstetricians have treated a
———————— baby in the breech position as an absolute reason for a caesarean, but this approach has been questioned and is not shared by all obstetricians. At issue here is the suggestion that breech babies born vaginally have a much greater risk of dying than babies in the cephalic (head-down) position. Against this must be weighed the fact that women are four times more likely to die from caesarean section than after a vaginal delivery.[19]

Before the 1970s, it was common practice for obstetricians to attempt to turn breech babies into the cephalic position, performing the procedure known as 'external cephalic version'. The increasing safety of the caesarean operation coupled with the fact that some babies turned back again into the breech position, or could not be turned into the cephalic position, led to a decline in this practice. With increasing concern about rising caesarean rates and the remaining risks of mortality or morbidity for the mother after caesarean section, some obstetricians are advocating a return of external cephalic version. It is now recommended that the procedure not be attempted until at least thirty-seven weeks of pregnancy to allow as much time as possible for a breech baby to turn spontaneously

....
19 Hofmeyr, 1991.

and for any other potential problems to become apparent. If the procedure itself then gives rise to problems (only a small risk), a mature baby could then be delivered by caesarean. Some obstetricians perform external cephalic version at forty weeks in the operating theatre of a labour ward to enable a swift caesarean operation, should this prove necessary.

Hofmeyr says that, at the most conservative estimate, attempted external cephalic version of all breech babies would prevent 34 per cent of breech deliveries and 14 per cent of caesareans for breech. He therefore recommends that women with breech babies be offered a choice of external cephalic version, vaginal delivery or elective caesarean with full information about the relative risks and benefits for both mother and baby. Another possibility is for a woman with a breech baby to use self-help methods for turning the baby such as special exercises.[20] Some acupuncturists and homoeopaths also claim to have been successful at encouraging breech babies to turn.

Mother's physical disability   When a woman has a physical disability which limits her mobility, it is common for some obstetricians to assume that she will deliver by caesarean. However, many physically disabled women are able to deliver vaginally and greatly value the opportunity to do so. One study, for example, showed that women with asthma were eighteen times more likely to have their condition exacerbated following a caesarean than after a vaginal delivery.[21] It is important for every woman to be viewed as an individual and for her potential for giving birth vaginally to be assessed objectively and communicated to her in an unbiased manner in order that she may make an informed choice about the manner of her baby's birth.

Repeat caesareans   The main concern is that as the caesarean rate rises for women having their first babies, the number of repeat caesareans will increase and become an important contribution to the overall rate. The majority of British obstetricians would allow a trial of labour following one caesarean and less than one in twenty subscribe to the traditional US view of 'once a caesarean, always a caesarean'. This is in fact an erroneous interpretation of Craigin's original lecture on the subject in 1916, when he pleaded for conservatism in the use of caesarean, which at that time was applied to 1 per cent of women.

....
20 Balaskas, 1989.
21 Mabie, Barton and Wasserstrumn, 1992.

He said that we should be cautious in performing the first caesarean as 'once a caesarean, always a caesarean'. In those days it was usually done for disproportion, so that was a reasonable expectation.

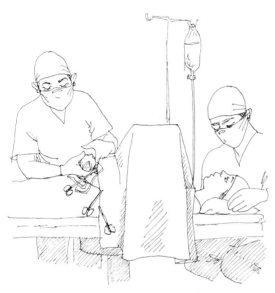

The reason that, until recently, American doctors continued to hold this view is that, in the case of about one in 200 women with a scar in the uterus, it will come apart (dehisce) during labour. Rarely, this may happen before labour starts. In a properly equipped hospital where it is possible to do a caesarean quickly, this rarely causes a problem for mother or child. This is discussed further in Chapter 9.

Classical (vertical) scars are considered more likely to rupture as the upper part (fundus) of the uterus is more muscular than the lower segment where the transverse incision is made. However, the classical incision was done commonly in the days when anaesthesia was not so advanced and blood transfusion and antibiotics were not available, so that rapid surgery and wound infection led to a higher chance of a weak scar. In 1968 in Kenya, Wendy Savage delivered a woman by caesarean of her thirteenth child which was too large to pass through her pelvis. In 1946 and 1947 her first two children had been born by caesarean and she then had ten normal deliveries. During the third operation the scar of the first could hardly be seen. This incident made Wendy Savage question the inherent weakness of these scars.

A new problem is vertical incisions in the lower segment. There is little evidence available about these and, just as in the United States some obstetricians are allowing women a trial of scar after two or more caesareans, so obstetricians should share their lack of knowledge and let the woman choose the manner of her delivery.

Apart from elective operations, a trial of scar can fail only because of the indications already given. Even repeat caesarean after two or more operations is unlikely to contribute more than another 0.5 per cent to the total rate.

CHAPTER SIX

The Modern Caesarean Operation: Coping with a Caesarean – for Parents, Midwives and Antenatal Teachers

If a woman is awake for the operation, every effort is usually made to explain to her and her labour companion what is going on and to make the experience as positive a one as possible.

In this chapter we discuss how to prepare for a caesarean; we describe what to expect during the procedure and after; we give advice to midwives caring for women after a caesarean; and throughout we present the sort of information that antenatal teachers might pass on to expectant parents.

PREPARATION FOR A CAESAREAN

The extent to which a woman can prepare for a caesarean depends in large part on whether it is an elective or an emergency operation. An elective caesarean is one which is planned in advance before the woman goes into labour. An emergency caesarean is usually performed during labour when the mother's or the baby's life may be considered to be at risk or when labour is not progressing. Many women having a caesarean may never have had an operation or general anaesthetic before, so they may have to come to terms with this as well as the fact that they will be giving birth by caesarean rather than vaginally.

Women having an elective caesarean can ask their doctor and midwife about the operation. They should be able to discuss the kind of anaesthetic to be used, whether their partner or labour companion can be present and any questions they may have about the procedure and their postnatal care. It is especially important to discuss what support will be available in hospital if a woman intends to breastfeed her baby. If a woman does not speak or understand English, it is essential that her midwife ensures that she has access to an interpreter or linkworker so that she can prepare for the operation.

Some women having an elective caesarean may feel uncomfortable about continuing to attend NHS or NCT antenatal classes. However, these are still valuable in order to enable women and their partners or labour companions to prepare for the birth and for life with a new baby. Breathing techniques for labour can help women remain calm if they are frightened at the prospect of the operation or if they are alarmed at the physical sensations often experienced during a caesarean. They also help with coughing and clearing the chest of secretions after a caesarean, particularly one under general anaesthetic. The relaxation techniques, as well as being skills useful for life in general, can help a woman cope with the caesarean itself, with post-operative pain and with breastfeeding.

Women and couples attending a well-run group often find the support from other members of their class invaluable. The midwife or antenatal teacher may be able to put them in touch with another woman or couple who have recently had a caesarean if they do not have a friend or relative who has had the same experience. Raising the subject at a class can also help prepare those women who may have an emergency caesarean, particularly if the chances of having a caesarean are presented in a realistic yet unalarming way.

> *At 36 weeks caesareans began to be mentioned and/or trial of labour. This was the hardest part, to decide what to do. I made contact with the local NCT and found a lady who had had the same problem. The hospital held a 'Caesar Evening' which was very helpful. I feel more information about caesareans should be given antenatally. For me it was not such a shock as I was able to find out so much beforehand.*[1]

Women expecting an elective caesarean have the opportunity to gear themselves up mentally for the operation. They can make arrangements in advance for practical support when they come home with the new baby, particularly if they have other children, and for the time when their partner, if they have one, may have gone back to work. It is also possible for women who use a homoeopath or herbalist to take advice about which remedies will aid their recovery after the operation. If a woman intends to breastfeed, it is important for her to let her midwives know and to have this written into her notes, particularly if she is having a general anaesthetic, as regrettably it is not yet assumed that a woman will breastfeed. She can also learn about the most comfortable positions

....
1 National Childbirth Trust, 1992.

for breastfeeding after the operation (see Further Information for Parents, page 198).

The preparations for an emergency caesarean are similar to those for an elective one, but everything happens faster. This can be bewildering for the woman, particularly if she does not understand English or is deaf, and so it is even more important that staff help by explaining to her and to her labour companion what is happening and the reasons for it. If the baby has become distressed, the woman will probably be asked to lie on her left side. This shifts the weight of the uterus away from the big blood vessels in her back. She may also be given oxygen to breathe through a mask. These are both ways of helping to give the baby more oxygen. The woman can use the breathing techniques learned for labour to keep calm.

Both before and during an emergency operation the woman's partner or other labour companion will have an important part to play in supporting the woman and helping her understand and come to terms with what is happening. This is particularly so if she is exhausted after a long labour or drowsy from the use of pain-killing drugs. The labour companion can take a photograph of the baby when it is first born and, if present during the operation, can describe the birth to the woman so she knows about the first few precious moments of her baby's life. If the labour companion is not present (often the case if a general anaesthetic is used), it is important that the woman's midwife or other member of staff present sees the woman after the operation to describe the birth and to answer any questions she may have. Sometimes it is possible for a member of staff or a student to take photographs. Doctors may not invite the labour companion into theatre, thinking that he or she may be shocked by the tubes going into the unconscious woman. If you want to be present, ask whether you can come in once the anaesthetist has done his or her job.

'I had nothing but praise for the sensitive way my emergency caesarean was handled – I was consulted then at every stage'.[2]

GOING INTO HOSPITAL

Women having an elective caesarean are usually admitted to hospital during the afternoon or evening before the operation. They can spend the time finding out about the postnatal ward to which they will go after the operation. They can begin to meet some of the midwives and feel a little more at home. Women who would rather spend the night at home may

2 National Childbirth Trust, 1992.

ask to come in on the day of the operation. This is often possible and a time is given after which the woman must not eat or drink anything if a general anaesthetic is planned or in case it should prove necessary.

It is important for the woman to be told what is happening at every stage, including who is responsible for her care (particularly after any change in shift), and to feel that she can ask about anything she needs to know.

CHOICE OF ANAESTHETIC

Our study of women's experiences revealed that 60 per cent of women were asleep for their caesarean but that the other 40 per cent were awake for the operation. Of the latter group, most women had an epidural block, while a few had a spinal block.

Because women have said that they missed the first precious moments of their baby's life, today many doctors advise women whenever possible to have a caesarean under epidural or spinal. The other disadvantages of a general anaesthetic are that:

- a woman may feel quite drowsy and disorientated for the first two or three days after delivery;
- the drugs may make the baby sleep and cause difficulties with breastfeeding;
- the woman's labour companion is not usually present during the operation, and may have to press to be allowed into the theatre.

However, some women prefer to be asleep for a caesarean and should feel able to ask for a general anaesthetic if that is the case.

The main advantages of an epidural anaesthetic for a caesarean are that:

- the woman can be conscious for the operation;
- her labour companion is normally invited to be present;
- the epidural can be used for more effective pain relief postnatally;
- the woman is easier to care for afterwards;
- the woman can put the baby to the breast earlier.

The main disadvantage of an epidural for caesarean is the small risk of a dural tap (see below).

When an emergency caesarean is necessary, there may or may not be time for an epidural to be administered but a spinal anaesthetic can be given. If a woman already has an epidural in place for routine pain relief, it can be 'topped up' with a larger dose of local anaesthetic to give the total pain relief necessary for abdominal surgery.

SPINAL BLOCK

A woman may be unable to have an epidural because there is insufficient time, or a general anaesthetic may be inadvisable for medical reasons or may be unacceptable to the woman. In these circumstances, the anaesthetist may be able to offer her a spinal block. A spinal block is a single injection of local anaesthetic given between two vertebrae in the lower spine (see illustration below), below the site of an epidural. A spinal block is quicker to perform and takes effect faster than an epidural, but lasts less time.

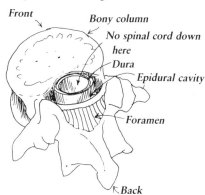

Line of episiotomy
Baby's head crowning

Front

Bony column

No spinal cord down here

Dura

Epidural cavity

Foramen

Back

Lower lumbar vertebra, 4 or 5

In the past, spinal block for caesarean was quite rare, possibly because of the risk of a severe headache afterwards from loss of spinal fluid following dural puncture. Now that the doctor uses a finer needle and the technique carries less risk of leakage, it is becoming more widely available. Because a spinal block can be performed only once, some anaesthetists also insert an epidural as the operation proceeds. This is in case anaesthesia is needed for longer than anticipated and also for administering pain relief after the operation.

In some hospitals, a spinal block is offered routinely instead of an epidural for both elective and emergency caesareans in order to save anaesthetists' time. Some women find that although they may experience more post-operative pain (because of the absence of the epidural tube for optimal pain relief), the quicker anaesthetic procedure makes the operation more acceptable.

PROCEDURE FOR ADMINISTERING AN EPIDURAL BLOCK

The woman must remain still for this skilled procedure, usually lying on her side or sitting on the side of the bed with her head bent forwards. After an injection of local anaesthetic has been given to numb the lower back, the anaesthetist inserts a needle closed with a stilette between two vertebrae in the lower back into the epidural space around the spinal cord (see illustration on page 78). Once the epidural space is identified, the stilette is withdrawn and a fine plastic tube is threaded through. The tube is taped securely to the woman's back and a small filter attached at the level of her shoulder. Some women find they have more sensation than others during the procedure: most do not feel anything, while others feel quite uncomfortable.

A test dose of local anaesthetic is given and, if all is well, the needle is withdrawn. Experienced anaesthetists may withdraw the needle before injecting the test dose. While the epidural is taking effect, the baby's heart rate is monitored continuously and a careful check kept on the woman's blood pressure in case it drops suddenly. An intravenous drip is always inserted into the woman's arm before the procedure in order that a serious fall in blood pressure (which can adversely affect the baby) may be corrected quickly.

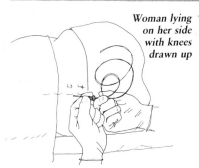

Woman lying on her side with knees drawn up

Introducing a catheter through a needle into the epidural space

There is a small risk of a dural tap when an epidural is inserted. This is when the needle goes in too far, punctures the protective sheath around the spinal cord and causes cerebrospinal fluid (the liquid that bathes the spinal cord and brain) to leak out. This can cause a woman to have a severe headache for several days. If a dural tap occurs, the woman is immediately asked to lie down. The headache is more severe when she sits up, so she is advised to lie down for as long as is necessary after the birth. This obviously makes life with a new baby much more difficult. Another more common problem is that the epidural does not work evenly or provide effective pain relief, so a general anaesthetic may be needed.

Some anaesthetists correct a dural tap by performing a 'blood patch'. This is done by drawing up some of the woman's blood into a needle and injecting the blood into the site of the dural tap. In many cases this prevents a headache. The risks of a dural tap are lower when an epidural is administered by an experienced anaesthetist skilled in the procedure.[3]

The operation is not allowed to start until the anaesthetist is satisfied that the anaesthetic is effective. This is tested by using a very cold spray or a sharp needle. Once the sensation of pain and cold are gone, the epidural is giving total pain relief.

PROCEDURE FOR ADMINISTERING A GENERAL ANAESTHETIC

One concern about general anaesthesia is that acid stomach contents may reach the lungs and cause problems. Most maternity units do not allow women

3 Personal communication to one of the authors.

to eat or drink once they are in the active phase of labour and some give regular doses of antacids routinely to all labouring women. There are differences of opinion among anaesthetists as to the best regimes. Prior to a general anaesthetic drugs may be given to neutralise or reduce the stomach contents.

The anaesthetic is introduced by means of a plastic cannula in the woman's arm. The drug passes into the bloodstream and leads to the woman being asleep in about thirty seconds. During this time the anaesthetist applies pressure to the woman's neck, pressing on the cricoid area to prevent any acid stomach contents reaching the lungs and causing damage. The anaesthetist next gives another injection which relaxes all the muscles. A tube is then introduced over the back of the throat and into the windpipe, after which the cricoid pressure can be released. The tube is then attached to a ventilator which breathes for the woman during the operation, ensuring she has the right amount of gas to keep her asleep and oxygen both for herself and the baby.

PROCEDURE FOR CAESAREAN SECTION

The woman will be wearing a hospital gown, will have removed any jewellery and contact lenses and may have had a little of her pubic hair shaved to clear the usual site of the caesarean section, slightly below the 'bikini line'. The woman's bladder is emptied by a catheter and some maternity units leave this in place until the next day. A soft metal plate is strapped around one of the woman's legs – this is the diathermy equipment – so that special forceps can be used to burn ('cauterise') small blood vessels in the wound and so control bleeding. A vertical metal screen is also positioned around the woman's waist to protect her from the diathermy. This, together with the liberal use of green sheets, means that the woman cannot see much of the operation even if she is awake for it. However, if she wishes, a mirror can be positioned to enable her to see what is going on.

The operating theatre, usually within the labour suite, contains the main operating table with large circular theatre lights above it. In addition there is a tray for resuscitating for the baby with a heater above it to keep the baby warm, a cot and an incubator, should it be needed.

There are usually four doctors present: an anaesthetist who will be at the mother's head; an obstetrician; an assistant; and a paediatrician who will check the baby after the birth. There are also several midwives including the 'scrub nurse', in charge of handing the instruments to the obstetrician, and the woman's midwife. In teaching hospitals there may be students and trainee anaesthetists as well. If a woman is awake for the operation, every effort is usually made to explain to her and her labour companion what is going on and to make the experience as positive a one as possible. Many women find that a cheerful and positive attitude on the part of the staff in the theatre makes the caesarean a less daunting experience than often anticipated.

'Thoughtful, constant listening care and an emergency caesarean, by epidural, which was more like a "party" than an operation'.[4]

All staff wash their hands thoroughly and wear sterile gowns and gloves. The anaesthetist will have ensured that the woman is sufficiently anaesthetised. He or she may use a needle or ice cube on different parts of the woman's abdomen to test for sensation. During the procedure some women feel nausea or dizziness (particularly after the baby is born). Oxygen can be administered through a small mask to alleviate this or anti-emetic/anti-sickness drugs are given. The woman's abdomen is exposed and cleaned with antiseptic solution, then sterile towels are draped over it, leaving only a small opening through which the operation will be performed.

To deliver a baby by caesarean, an incision is made first in the wall of the abdomen and is generally about 5 or 6 inches long. This is usually horizontal and sometimes called the 'bikini cut'. Only if the baby is in a transverse position or if there is placenta praevia or some other medical reason is a vertical incision made these days. Even if the woman has a previous vertical scar, a horizontal incision may be used to make post-operative recovery more rapid. Even with good regional anaesthesia, a caesarean can be full of sensation for the woman, who may panic if she is not prepared for this and wonders what she might feel next. If she hates the sensations and finds that she cannot cope with being awake for the operation, she should tell the anaesthetist and, if she prefers, ask to have a general anaesthetic. Women have reported feeling 'as if someone were drawing on your skin with a pencil', 'feeling slightly tickly' or 'a sharp pain over the pubic bone' as the obstetrician made the first incision. Pain sensation is more easily abolished than stretching feelings.

It normally takes only five to ten minutes to deliver the baby. The uterus is in the middle of the abdomen with the bowels above and behind. The bladder lies over the lower part of the uterus and is pushed down so that the obstetrician can reach the thinner lower segment of the uterus. A second horizontal incision is made in the lower segment of the uterus. Both incisions are cauterised to minimise blood loss. Women have reported a 'sensation of wet' as the warm amniotic fluid runs down

4 National Childbirth Trust, 1992.

between their legs after the second incision. An electric pump is used to suck out the amniotic fluid and any blood from the uterus; some parents comment on the 'slurping' noises. The doctor's hand then reaches deep into the uterus and delivers the baby through the opening. If the baby is head down, the doctor may be able to cup a hand under the head and lift it through the opening, but sometimes small forceps are used instead. Once the head is through, the rest of the baby's body slips out easily in a similar manner to a vaginal birth. A woman who is awake for the operation may feel a variety of sensations as the baby is delivered, but should feel no pain. Women have described sensations as if someone were 'rummaging around the bottom of a drawer' or a 'shopping bag'. The baby usually splutters and gasps and may cry. The umbilical cord is clamped and cut immediately. The paediatrician will normally want to check the baby and suck out any fluid from its nose and mouth. The doctor will then deliver the placenta and membranes. If the woman has not been in labour (as in an elective caesarean), the cervix is stretched open from inside the uterus to allow drainage (of blood etc.) into the vagina.

Under general anaesthetic, the level given to the woman during the birth is relatively light so that the baby is not born too drowsy. Because of this, women sometimes have an awareness of voices or things happening but there is no sensation of pain. After the baby is born, the level of anaesthetic is increased and the much longer process of putting the uterus and abdominal wall back together again begins. This usually takes about thirty to fifty minutes. Dissolving sutures are used to sew the wound in the uterus. The final layer of the skin is nowadays usually closed by a continuous hidden stitch kept in place by beads at either end or by staples which are removed after four or five days, when the outside of the wound has healed. Sometimes it may be beneficial for the doctor to remove any blood collected in the wound with a small plastic drain coming from the side of the wound and leading into a small glass bottle. The wound is covered either by spraying on a plastic protective layer, or with gauze and sticking plaster or similar sticky tape.

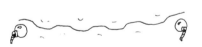

Running stitch under the skin, fixed with beads

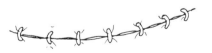

Wound clipped together with curved staples

After the birth, the woman is given an injection of syntometrine to minimise the risk of heavy bleeding from the uterus (postpartum haemorrhage) and the baby is given vitamin K. After a caesarean under general anaesthetic, the woman is transferred to the recovery room where she is brought round and shown the baby. It is common for women to fall asleep again and to wake up on the postnatal ward wondering what has happened. If the woman's labour companion can stay with the woman until she wakes up again, this can be very helpful.

THE SCAR

The modern lower-segment caesarean section gives a stronger scar than a classical vertical one. It heals more quickly and easily, causes less discomfort to the woman during recovery and should withstand any future labour contractions. Occasionally, if there are problems with a lower-segment operation, for example if a large fibroid is obstructing access, then a vertical incision is made in the thicker and more muscular upper segment of the uterus. A vertical or 'classical' incision may also be performed for transverse lie or placenta praevia. What the doctor wants to avoid is a T-shaped incision which is thought to be the weakest scar of all.

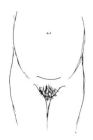
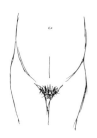

'Bikini' line cut   *Vertical cut*

It is important for subsequent births that women should know the type of scar they have on their uterus. A vertical scar is more likely to tear in labour than a horizontal one. However, a vertical scar on the abdomen does not necessarily mean a vertical scar on the uterus which will usually have a horizontal segment scar. If the woman does not know what type of scar she has, the doctor can usually feel a transverse scar, during a vaginal examination in early labour.

CARE AFTER A CAESAREAN

Some hospitals have single rooms available to which women who have had caesareans are given priority. Other hospitals have 'amenity rooms': private rooms for which NHS patients may pay in order to have this privacy. Many women find the relative peace and quiet of a room to themselves makes a positive difference to the first few days of their recovery.

'I feel very strongly that after such a bad time (my surgeon's own words) I should have been put in an amenity room . . . and I would have willingly paid but I was in no fit state to ask and it did not occur to my poor hus-

band ... it would certainly have aided my recovery'.[5]

If a baby dies, it may seem even harder that, despite having a caesarean, this has happened. A woman in this situation needs both a great deal of time to talk through the experience and sensitive support on the lines recommended by SANDS (see Further Information for Parents, page 198).

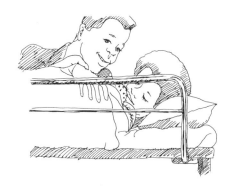

PAIN RELIEF   It is important for the woman to be made comfortable so that she can become mobile as soon as possible and feel able to feed and get to know her baby, particularly in the first twenty-four hours after birth when the post-operative pain is at its highest level. If the woman has had an epidural and staffing levels on the postnatal ward are adequate, the tube will be left in for twenty-four hours, because this is the most effective method of administering pain relief. Otherwise, the woman is given injections of pain-relieving drugs into her bottom or thigh. Once the woman is able to drink, she can change from injections to pain-relieving tablets. Some hospitals give a cocktail of soluble pain-killer with peppermint water for wind and an antacid for heartburn. The pain-relieving drugs used are safe for breastfeeding mothers to take as the amounts transferred to the baby are minimal. It is therefore better to have adequate relief from pain and discomfort than to try to manage without. Some women use the TENS machine they have hired for labour for post-operative pain relief. TENS is believed to have no side-effects on mother or baby, but this has not yet been scientifically evaluated. Equally, natural therapies are considered by some people to be helpful at this time, but they too have not been evaluated. Some women cope with the pain of removing sticking plaster from the site of the drip in their arm and the wound by gently loosening it themselves.

MOBILITY AND CARING FOR THE BABY   The art of recovering after a caesarean is in maintaining a balance between gradually becoming mobile and being able to care for the baby with having enough opportunities for rest and not becoming exhausted by doing too much too soon. It is vital that

....

5 National Childbirth Trust, 1992.

sufficient practical support and help in hospital is easily available. Having to ask repeatedly for help increases some women's feelings of inadequacy so that either help should be offered or women should be made to feel free to ask for it. Women have the right to this sort of support and should not feel that it reflects adversely on them if they need it. It is important for the woman to have early access to a physiotherapist to show her how to guard her wound and become mobile. Any breathing and relaxation techniques she has learned for labour will be useful at this time.

Women are encouraged to get out of bed and begin caring for their baby as soon as possible because this improves blood circulation and aids recovery. It may seem cruel to make a woman get up on the first day after an operation, but with a lower-segment scar and with good pain relief it is often possible and may be beneficial for a woman's morale as well as her physical well-being. While in bed it is important for the woman to keep her legs moving by circling her ankles and wriggling her toes. This improves circulation and prevents blood clots. Some women are given injections to help thin the blood until they are fully mobile. If the woman has had a caesarean after a trial of forceps or Ventouse, her perineum may feel stiff and sore and she may need a rubber ring or special inflatable cushion (available for hire from local NCT branches if not available from the NHS) to sit on.

At first, the woman may need some help to get out of bed and sit on a chair and later to walk to the lavatory. It helps to keep her bed as low as possible and a monkey bar may also be used so that the woman can pull herself up. Getting out of bed will take time and the woman should try to find the most comfortable way for herself. One way is for her to sit up and gradually shuffle her bottom sideways to the edge of the bed, pushing her hands into the bed to help her lift her bottom. She can then lower one leg at a time on to the floor and swivel her body so that she is sitting

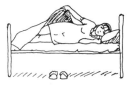

1. Roll onto one side

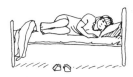

2. Knees up, top hand across onto the bed

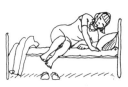

3. Push on top hand, swing feet down gently

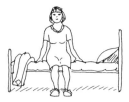

4. Feet apart, push up on both hands

Getting out of bed without hurting yourself

on the edge of the bed. When she is ready, she can gently move into a chair or get up and walk (see illustrations on page 84).

The woman may be surprised at the length of time she needs to get up and walk to the lavatory; she may need someone with her for reassurance and to make sure she is all right. She should allow herself as much time as she needs for getting out of bed, then for standing up. She should not walk until she is standing up straight and should be encouraged to stand as upright as possible, since this aids recovery, as well as her self-respect. Then she can look ahead and think about moving. To walk, she can lean her weight on one foot, then swing the other leg forward, shift her weight to that foot and repeat the movement: by using the momentum of her legs in this way, she puts less strain on the wound.

If the woman's baby is in a special care baby unit (SCBU) without beds for mothers, or even in a different hospital, it is vital that staff enable her to see the baby as soon as possible. She can be taken in a wheelchair to see the baby. Even if the woman is unable to feed the baby herself, she can let the baby hear her voice and feel her touch which can be a positive experience for them both. Usually a photograph is taken and given to her to help her cope with the interval before seeing her baby.

GOING TO THE LAVATORY   As mentioned above, some maternity units leave a catheter in place for the first twenty-four hours to drain the bladder. Otherwise the woman can use a bedpan or ask the midwives to sit her on a commode. If the woman cannot empty her bladder, her midwife may need to insert a catheter to relieve the pressure and prevent the bladder becoming overstretched. After the first night, the woman should be feeling well enough to make her way to the lavatory.

It is very common for women to have a lot of wind after a caesarean, as with any other abdominal operation. This can be uncomfortable, so the woman should be encouraged to pass any wind and to avoid fizzy drinks, including carbonated mineral water. Peppermint water can help with the problem.

The woman is unlikely to open her bowels on the first day but if, as can happen, she becomes constipated, she may wish to take gentle laxatives or suppositories to keep the motions soft and avoid straining. If a woman is breastfeeding, there are certain kinds of laxative she should avoid. Fibre-rich foods can help: some women take dried apricots as a snack in their hospital bag. Occasionally, certain kinds of pain-killing drugs can cause constipation and alternatives should be used.

FOOD AND DRINK   The intravenous drip is normally kept in place for twelve to twenty-four hours after birth to ensure the woman receives enough liquid. In addition, the woman is given mouthwashes and small amounts of water which are gradually increased. Care should be taken to avoid increasing the liquid intake too fast which may cause the mother to feel sick. Once the woman can drink freely, the drip can be removed. When she is drinking normally and bowel sounds are present, she can start eating solid foods, building up initially from a light diet.

COUGHING   It is important for the woman to cough and clear phlegm from her chest after the operation, especially if she has had a general anaesthetic. If she smokes, the problem can be worse and she could be at risk of a chest infection. A physiotherapist will help her cough and it may be useful to her to have some pain relief before the physiotherapy. The physiotherapist will teach the woman how to support her scar with her hands when she coughs. This is also helpful when she laughs or uses the lavatory.

SLEEP   At first the woman will be propped up in bed to sleep and pain-killing injections or tablets will help. It is very important that the woman's sleep is not disturbed by pain. It used to be the practice for the baby to be taken to the nursery in order for the woman to get an undisturbed night's rest. However, many women intending to breastfeed prefer to keep their baby with them all the time and in some maternity units nurseries are no longer used. Where there is a hospital nursery, some women find it helpful the first two nights after the birth for the staff to change and settle the baby, bringing the baby to the woman just for breastfeeding, so that she gets as much rest as possible. If a woman does have her baby with her, it is essential for her calls for assistance to be answered within a reasonable time if the baby needs to be lifted out of the cot for feeding or comforting. The woman should be encouraged to try to sleep whenever the opportunity presents itself, particularly if she has been woken in the night for feeds.

BREASTFEEDING   *'I was given great help with feeding the baby following the caesarean section despite the fact I had previously successfully breastfed both children.'*
    'I cannot praise highly enough the sister on the ward who spent hours (literally) with myself and the baby. At every feed she would be there

encouraging the baby to latch on and she refused to give in'.[6]

It is now accepted that the vast majority of women are physically capable of breastfeeding (97 per cent according to World Health Organization figures). The superiority of breastmilk has led to the recommendation that all babies should be exclusively breastfed for the first four to six months.[7] Therefore breastfeeding after a caesarean is to be recommended, not only because it is best for the baby, but also because it helps the uterus return to its normal size more quickly. The fact that the woman has had an abdominal operation may make breastfeeding more uncomfortable than after a vaginal delivery, but there are many ways in which she can adapt to the situation. What is important is that the people around her support her in her wish to breastfeed and help her remain confident in her ability to do so.

Some women are able to breastfeed immediately after the operation if they are not too drowsy or if they have had an epidural or spinal block. This gives the mother and the baby a chance to be especially close and may give the woman a feeling of normality at being able to feed the baby herself, particularly if she is disappointed at having had a caesarean. There is usually plenty of time while the obstetrician is repairing the wound. Some women ask for the baby to be put to the breast while they are still asleep under the general anaesthetic. Another way of caring for the baby during this time is for the father or other labour companion to cuddle the baby next to their skin.

The woman will need help getting into a comfortable position so that the baby can feed without resting on the wound. This can be achieved by the woman either sitting up or lying down. Hospital beds are not ideal places to breastfeed, so she may need to experiment to find comfortable positions, with pillows and lots of help. If the woman needs to be propped upright following a general anaesthetic, she will need help with pillows to be able to feed in a good position without pulling the breast out of the baby's mouth. The back-rest of the bed should be in its upright position with a pillow across her lap and the baby resting on the pillow; or the pillow can be at her side and the baby lying on the pillow with its feet tucked under her arm (also known as the 'football hold' or 'underarm position'). Another way for the baby to feed in hospital is lying on a pillow on the meal table which fits over the bed. Alternatively the woman could sit on a chair with her feet up on a stool to keep her legs higher than her wound. If the woman lies on her side, the baby can

....

6 National Childbirth Trust, 1992.
7 Royal College of Midwives, 1991.

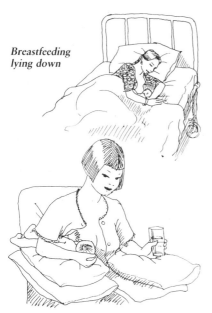

*Breastfeeding
lying down*

*Breastfeeding well
supported in an upright
chair*

lie on his side next to her (see illustrations).

Latching the baby correctly onto the breast is very important for all breastfeeding and the mother will be helped at first by the midwives to achieve this. The baby needs to be facing the mother, lying on his side, with his mouth close to the nipple. His mouth needs to be open really wide, with the bottom lip curled back. When he is correctly positioned, his chin will be tucked into the breast, with a really good amount of breast tissue in his mouth. Most of the areola, particularly the underside, will be in his mouth, although just how much depends on the individual woman. The mother should not attempt to shape the breast with her hand in order to help the baby fix on. If she feels that the breast needs support, she should support it from below, with the flat of her hand against her rib-cage.

If the baby is latched on well, the top of his ears may wiggle and the muscles at the temples may move as well. He will suck quickly at first, and then, as the milk lets down, he will change to slower, deeper and more rhythmic sucks, often accompanied by gulping noises. The mother should be encouraged to let the baby finish the first breast by himself to make sure that he gets as much of the higher-fat hind-milk as possible. She can then offer the second side if he wants it.

It is vital that the woman receives plenty of support from her midwives in learning how to latch on the baby correctly. Since they will have to lift the baby out of the cot for her, this should not be a problem. The midwives should also help the woman change to the other breast when the baby has finished on the first side, although often the baby will have fallen asleep and come off the breast, having had a satisfying feed from just the one side. If feeding becomes uncomfortable, the woman can remove the baby from the breast gently by putting her little finger into the corner of his mouth to break the suction, before encouraging him to latch on correctly before feeding again. In time the woman and baby will learn good positioning together.

Breathing and relaxation techniques learned for labour are good for breastfeeding too, and the woman can be reminded to use them if she forgets. One of the things to be aware of during the early days of breastfeeding after a caesarean is that the pain-killing drugs may cause the pain of a poorly latched-on baby or of sore nipples not to be apparent. It is also possible for a drowsy baby to drift off to sleep during feeds, slide off the nipple a bit, wake up and then start feeding again in a poor position which is likely to cause damage to the nipple. It is therefore important for the woman and her midwives together to try to ensure that the baby always feeds correctly positioned.

Sometimes women who have had a caesarean find that it takes longer for the breastmilk to come in after the colostrum. If this is the case, the woman should not be allowed to lose confidence in her ability to feed the baby. Although the anaesthetics used for caesareans have not been shown to be the cause of such a delay, it is thought that there are factors which do not help. These might include the fact that the woman may have been without food and drink for as long as two or three days. Other reasons might be a drowsy baby feeding less often and sucking less strongly than a more alert baby, and a woman reluctant to put the baby to the breast as frequently as a woman who does not have an abdominal scar to contend with.

The woman should be encouraged to feed the baby with colostrum whenever he shows signs of being hungry so as to help the milk come in. Sometimes midwives offer to give the baby a bottle to allow the mother an opportunity to rest, particularly during the night. However, giving bottles of water, dextrose or formula will only serve to delay the milk for longer by depriving the woman's breasts of the stimulation they need from the baby's sucking. It has been shown that supplementary and complementary feeds may ultimately reduce the time a woman breastfeeds her baby.[8] If the milk is delayed for as long as five or six days, as can happen sometimes, it is important for the woman not to lose heart and to remember that colostrum is a valuable food, richer in calories and antibodies than breastmilk. It may be that her system is taking longer to get under way, but the baby will not suffer and her milk will come in eventually.

In order to make breastfeeding as easy as possible, the woman should wear a front-opening nightdress or a loose T-shirt which can be pulled up and a proper nursing bra for good support of the breasts.

If the woman's baby is in a SCBU, the woman will need even more support for breastfeeding, particularly if he is premature or sick. If the baby is unable to breastfeed at all or for long enough to get sufficient nourishment, the

....

8 Royal College of Midwives, 1991, p. 41.

woman will need to be shown how to use an electric breastpump to help establish and maintain her milk supply. The expressed milk can then be fed to the baby by tube. This can help the woman feel that she is doing something positive for the baby which no one else can do. Skin-to-skin contact helps stimulate the milk-producing hormones as well as enabling the woman to be especially close to her baby. Support from an NCT breastfeeding counsellor can be particularly valuable in this situation. Specialist leaflets are available for mothers who have had caesareans and for those whose babies are in special care, giving practical information on expressing and storing breastmilk (see Further Information for Parents, page 198).

WASHING   It is probably best to wait a day for the first wash and then to give the mother a bedbath, of course keeping away from the area of the wound. After this, the woman will probably be able to wash herself and a shower may be easiest if she finds bending over very painful. It is important for the woman to keep the wound as clean and dry as possible to promote healing and prevent infection. If she has a bath in hospital or uses a bidet, it is essential that these are cleaned before use with a disinfectant or cream cleanser and her own cleaning cloth. The seat of the lavatory and bidet can be cleaned using antiseptic wipes. If the woman is unfortunate enough to have had stitches in her perineum as well (from an episiotomy for trial of forceps or Ventouse), these will also have to be kept especially clean and dry. A hairdrier is not recommended for drying stitches.

THE WOUND   As mentioned above, sometimes a small plastic drain will be used to take away into a small glass bottle any blood that might have congealed. It is usually removed the day after the operation by gently pulling it out. The elastic top of normal briefs may chafe the wound, a situation which may last for many months, so it is usually better for the woman to wear knickers that come up to her waist and to avoid sanitary belts which may rub. The soft, stretchy briefs sold by NCT (Maternity Sales) Limited are ideal as they are elastic enough to hold a sanitary pad in place and to stop any chafing of stitches in the perineum (see Further Information for Parents, page 198). Loose, comfortable clothes which do not press on the wound are essential.

   There are several ways of closing the caesarean wound in the abdomen. Some stitches are hidden and dissolve so that there is nothing to remove later. Others are hidden but do not dissolve. These are fixed at either end of the wound with a small bead and are easily (and fairly painlessly) removed by cutting one bead free and pulling the other with the thread out of the wound. Alternatively there may be individual stitches, clips and/or staples to remove. In the case of a horizontal cut the stitches will be removed after four or five days, but with a vertical cut they will be left in for seven to ten days.

Some women suffer because the wound becomes infected; it looks red and inflamed and may be painful. This can be helped by making a small hole in the wound with a probe and taking out the pus. A poultice or heat pad placed over the wound may also help to draw out the pus. It is vital to keep the wound as clean and dry as possible. The wound will remain quite sensitive for a while. As it heals, its colour changes from red to brown to white, by which time it will probably be covered by the pubic hair which will have grown in again. It may become itchy and this can be eased with a light vegetable oil. It is not uncommon for women to feel numbness around the scar. This sensation may last for several months and in fact a small area may remain permanently numb.

BLEEDING FROM THE VAGINA ('LOCHIA') This is the same as after a vaginal delivery. The lochia is red at first, but after about five days will change to a brown colour and resemble the discharge at the end of a period. It will finally change to a watery yellow-brown or pink discharge. Many women who breastfeed find that after a feed they experience 'after-pains' when the oxytocin released by the baby's suckling causes the uterus to contract down and a little fresh blood may be found on the sanitary pad shortly after. This is quite normal and the woman will usually be able to deal with the discharge by using sanitary pads. However, she should be advised to tell her midwife if the bleeding becomes heavier, begins to smell offensive or if she passes blood clots. This could indicate an infection in the uterus or that a piece of the placenta or membranes is still inside the uterus. This can be checked using ultrasound and, if necessary, the woman will be taken to theatre and, under general anaesthetic, the uterus is gently scraped until it is empty.

INFECTIONS It is possible that the woman may get an infection in her urine, chest, breasts, wound or uterus. If the woman has a persistently high temperature, her doctor will check her for any site of infection and she may need to take antibiotics. These may make the woman feel rather tired and may lead to diarrhoea. If the woman is breastfeeding, the baby's stools may become even looser than is usual with breastfeeding, but this does not usually cause a problem provided that the woman is warned that it may happen. In some hospitals, women are given antibiotics at delivery as a preventative measure against infection.

VISITORS On the first day after the caesarean, it is probably best if the woman sees as few people as possible so that she can rest. She will probably want to see her partner and other children and will find their support with becoming mobile and caring for the baby helpful. But the woman may want to keep other visitors to a minimum so that she can use her time in hospital to rest and recover as much as she can before going home. It is important for the woman's partner to be aware of her need for support and, when telling family and friends about the new baby, to ask them not to visit until the woman is ready to appreciate their company.

When the woman goes home, it may be necessary to ration visitors then too, particularly if they make her feel she has to rush around tidying up and cleaning and making cups of tea. On the other hand, visitors who come with food and to help with chores may be very welcome!

COPING AT HOME Nowadays, as the result of the quicker healing of the horizontal caesarean scar, most women stay in hospital for only five days rather than the ten-day period which was usual in the past. Women usually go home when the stitches have been removed from the wound, at about five days. In some areas women go home after four days if all is well and they feel ready, and the community midwife removes the stitches on the fifth day.

All women who have had a caesarean need practical support until they have recovered fully from what is, after all, major abdominal surgery. Therefore all genuine offers of help should be accepted, particularly if there are other children and the woman's partner has to go back to work a few days after her return home. Some women have a relative or friend to stay and help or have their friends and neighbours look after the children, do the shopping and drop in with food they have cooked. Other women stay with their mother or other relative so that they can be looked after. Women who are alone or who have difficulties with coping at home may need the practical help and support of a home help or family aide. Either the community midwife or health visitor can make suitable arrangements; if things are very difficult, they can arrange for the support of a social worker. When the community midwife transfers care of the woman to a health visitor, good communication about the caesarean and any other relevant factors is of paramount importance.

Some health professionals arrange for this handover of care to take place with the woman present, so that she can be involved too.

It is important in the first couple of weeks at home that the woman is free to concentrate solely on her own rest and recovery and on feeding and caring for the baby. During the first two weeks after birth, babies often sleep a lot as they too recover from the birth and start getting used to the world outside the uterus.

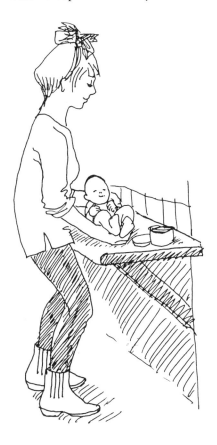

This is a good time for the woman to rest as much as she can so that when after two weeks the baby is awake for longer each day and therefore needs to feed more often, she will be able to cope more easily. Some women find the support of a breastfeeding counsellor from the NCT helpful if they need extra help with breastfeeding.

Gradually, the woman will be able to take on her normal duties at home. Heavy lifting must be avoided for at least six weeks. Women are also advised not to drive for six weeks in case an emergency stop puts a sudden strain on the scar. A couple can start having penetrative sex again whenever they both feel ready. However, a woman cannot have a coil or other inter-uterine contraceptive device fitted until three months after the birth instead of the usual six weeks.

EMOTIONS   *'All the midwives in the hospital and afterwards were very kind and prepared to listen, but when I was in the depths of despair, (after the operation and later at home) perhaps I could have benefited from someone trained in counselling who would know the right questions to ask.'*[9]

Some women find the emotional aftermath of a caesarean to be of more significance to them than its physical aspects. The resulting emotions and

....

9 National Childbirth Trust, 1992.

thoughts are likely to carry on for longer than the physical recovery and, in some cases, may not even begin until the woman starts to get back to normal. Immediately after any birth the woman's feelings towards her baby are likely to be volatile. They may swing from immense maternal love at one extreme to indifference and feelings of unreality. Studies have shown that about 40 per cent of mothers find that the elation and love for the baby they expected to feel immediately after the birth in fact took several days to develop.

If the caesarean came after a long and difficult labour, the woman may be glad that it is all over and be delighted with her baby. However, her tiredness and feelings of relief may be so strong that there is no room for other emotions. In order to help the woman relate to her baby, she can be encouraged to hold and examine the baby as soon as possible after the birth. If the baby is dried, it will not lose heat so quickly if the woman wants to take her time. The first feed at the breast is a good way of establishing contact, whenever the woman and baby are ready. Even if the baby does not want to feed at first, being held close will enable the baby to smell, taste and feel its mother as well as recognise her voice. Skin-to-skin contact will also help to stimulate the woman's milk supply. As with any birth, the baby will be getting used to life outside the uterus with its bright lights, loud sounds and intriguing sights.

It is common for nearly all women to experience the 'baby blues' on the third or fourth day after birth. The woman may find herself crying for no reason and she may also be irritable, anxious, forgetful, confused and disorientated. She may fear rejection by her partner. All new parents have concerns about the well-being of their baby and worry that it may not be all right. However, some women may become excessively anxious for no reason and be suspicious that there are things about the baby that they have not been told. Birth may revive unconscious memories and feelings about siblings or herself which may contribute to the woman's distress.

There are other ways in which the baby blues become evident. They may last for only a day but in other cases for a couple of weeks. Ten per cent of women experience postnatal depression, a clinical problem which may need professional help, as well as understanding and support from their family and friends. Postnatal depression is more common after a caesarean than a vaginal delivery. This is due, at least in part, to the fact that in addition to recovering from dramatic changes in hormone levels, the woman is recovering from a major operation with physical discomfort, tiredness and possible infection to compound the usual problems of getting used to feeding and caring for a new baby. It can be depressing for the woman to keep asking for help, to see other women get back to 'normal' more quickly after vaginal deliveries and to find that not everyone is sympathetic. In addition there may be feelings of inadequacy and disappointment at not having had the kind of birth that was planned. Some women feel that they were at fault and that they are not a 'real woman'. This may be compounded in some ethnic groups by negative attitudes towards caesarean section by the partner or community.[10] For most women, these feelings will pass fairly quickly, but other women will need extra help and understanding in coming to terms with them.

It is important to see that the woman is given space and time to express her feelings. Before she leaves hospital, her midwives and doctors should ensure that she has had an opportunity to discuss the birth and ask questions. All women appreciate visits during their stay in hospital from the professionals who cared for them during labour and this is even more the case for women who have had a difficult labour or a caesarean. In some instances, it may be appropriate to offer the woman a follow-up appointment at the time of the routine six-week postnatal check or at some other time if there are still unresolved issues. Alternatively, the woman may welcome the opportunity to talk over the birth with an obstetric counsellor or member of the psychiatric staff at the hospital. After traumatic deliveries a few women feel that they lost control of their labour and report feelings akin to those of women who have been raped. Deep-rooted feelings do not respond to reassurance and women who have them may require professional psychological support beyond simply talking through the experience.

The woman's partner, if she has one, will have an important role to play, as will her family and friends. Any woman, whatever her situation, may benefit from a talk with her midwife, health visitor, GP or a social worker. For women keen to meet other local mothers with new babies, there are informal postnatal support groups as well as special caesarean support groups run by women which can be contacted through their health visitor, local branches of the NCT or through the Caesarean Support Network (see Further Information for Parents, page 198).

....
10 Savage, 1986, p. 160.

CHAPTER SEVEN

WOMEN'S EXPERIENCE OF CAESAREANS

Obviously any woman would prefer a normal delivery,
but an elective section using a spinal or epidural
anaesthetic is the next best thing. A caesarean birth can
be a very positive and moving experience and with
post-operative pain relief can easily be coped with.

IT is women who give birth and who cope with the after-effects, but little research is done into their feelings and opinions about their care. We therefore felt that it was very important to ask women about their experiences, feelings and reactions following a caesarean operation. The women were contacted through nine hospitals randomly selected to represent the populations in different health authority regions across the country and data were collected from 300 women. Details of the methodology of the survey and tables of the results appear in Appendices B and C.

REASONS FOR CAESAREAN SECTION

The mothers were asked: 'What reason(s) did the doctors give for performing a caesarean operation? You may have been given more than one reason so please tick the answers that apply to you.' There followed a list of 'reasons' and space for women to add any explanations given to them that were not included in the list. The results were tabulated (Table A1, page 180) and show that women were told that caesarean sections were necessary because of a combination of factors. Some women were given as many as three or four reasons and others only one. The proportion of reasons given by women who had emergency rather than elective caesareans differed greatly.

Elective caesareans

A recent study where the reasons given by women were checked against case notes showed that most women knew why they had had a caesarean.[1] The results of our survey show that four out of five women who had an elective caesarean had it for three reasons: previous caesareans, size of pelvis in relation to size

---

1 Hillan, 1992b.

of the baby, and breech presentation. Over half (56.8 per cent) of the elective operations were carried out because women had had previous caesareans. Two in five women (41.7 per cent) were told that their babies were too big for vaginal delivery and almost three out of ten women (28.8 per cent) were operated on because their babies were in the breech position. 'Other' reasons specified by women for their elective operations included their age (3 per cent) and the existence of fibroids (2.3 per cent). Neither of these reasons were mentioned by women having emergency operations, presumably because such factors were determined antenatally. Fewer women had elective caesareans for unstable fetal position, previous problems with vaginal delivery, placenta praevia and transverse lie.

Emergency caesareans The two main reasons were that labour was taking a long time and that the baby was distressed. These accounted for almost half (49.1 per cent) of all reasons for emergency caesareans. This highlights a very large difference between the elective and emergency caesarean groups in that only 1.9 per cent of elective operations were done for fetal distress as compared with 36.3 per cent of emergency ones. But of course, elective caesareans are decided upon before labour begins. The third most common reason given for emergency sections was that the baby was too big for the woman's pelvis. Nearly one in five (18.5 per cent) were told this. Attempts to determine antenatally whether the pelvis is too small for the baby have been unsuccessful — even when X-ray pelvimetry was used to measure the size of the bony pelvis, instead of clinical assessment. Estimating the size of the baby by ultrasound or clinical palpation is also imprecise.

Two in five (42.3 per cent) of the women having an emergency section were told that labour was taking too long and almost the same number (36.3 per cent) were told that their baby was in distress. Clearly when labour is prolonged, the woman gets tired and the baby may become distressed as its reserves of glycogen are used up, so it is not surprising that some women mentioned both reasons. Other reasons given to women for their emergency caesareans included high blood pressure (4.1 per cent), maternal distress (1.5 per cent) and protein in the urine (1.1 per cent).

WOMEN'S REQUEST FOR CAESAREAN SECTION In an attempt to find out whether the use of caesarean section was due to doctors responding to women's requests, mothers were asked: 'Did you ask to have a caesarean section?' The results show that almost one woman in seven (13.2 per cent) asked for one. There were great differences in the percentage according to whether the woman was having her first baby or because of her previous experience of childbirth. One in five (21.9 per cent) of the women who had had a caesarean for their first delivery asked for another. This contrasts with only one in twelve (8 per cent) of those having their first baby. Over half (53.8 per cent) of the women requesting the operation had had previous caesareans. From the fact that almost one in seven women said they requested a caesarean, it is surprising that this reason did not emerge more prominently in the consultants' survey. Less than one in fifty mentioned it as a factor. However, this may be because women asked for a caesarean which their obstetrician had not recommended.

Women who requested a caesarean were asked why they had done so. Many of those for whom this was not the first caesarean said that they had requested the operation because the original reasons for the previous caesarean were still valid. Others stressed their desire to pre-empt the need for an emergency caesarean. Some of the comments were as follows:

'I didn't want to go through labour and end up having a section like last time.'

'I anticipated I would need one and did not want another emergency operation.'

'Elective is by far preferable to emergency.'

Others had requested caesareans because of concern for their babies, presumably based on their previous experiences:

'I didn't want to put baby in distress.'

'I feel it's the safest option for the child.'

'I had a fear of the baby being in trouble again.'

Similarly those women who had previously given birth vaginally but had requested a caesarean for this birth stated reasons to do with their past experience(s), for example:

'I had a previous difficult delivery.'

Only a few women having their first child requested a caesarean. These were more often than not done as an emergency after a trial of labour.

'I was in constant pain for hours and felt that I couldn't go on any longer.'

One woman stated that she had requested the operation because of her 'Very painful labour'. Another said she had asked for a caesarean because '*I was told that forceps would be necessary and I would not agree to their use*'.

So some women do want a caesarean, but seven out of eight (86.8 per cent) women having one agreed to the procedure on the advice of medical practitioners.

BEING AWAKE FOR Women were asked: 'During the operation
THE CAESAREAN were you awake or asleep?' The results showed
that overall three in five (60.3 per cent) of the women were asleep during their operation. However, three-quarters (75 per cent) of the women having emergency sections were asleep during the operation compared to only two in five of those having elective caesareans. It is surprising that over two out of five (41.7 per cent) of the women receiving elective caesareans had them under general anaesthetic despite the fact that, presumably, the woman would have had an element of control over what happened to her and the emergency situation did not apply.

This position could be explained in a number of ways. It may be hospital policy which dictates whether or not a woman is allowed to be awake during the operation. Another possibility is that a suitably skilled anaesthetist was not available to perform an epidural. From the comments it does not seem that the expectant mothers wanted to be asleep. Information from mothers also reflected their lack of preparation for operative birth and lack of information about what would happen to them. Some relevant comments were as follows:

'*I found a planned section with epidural a far more pleasant and positive experience than my first section which was an emergency with general anaesthetic after a very long labour. My first section was a distressing and frightening experience and one which I felt completely unprepared for.*'

'*Although I understand that the well-being of my baby was of paramount importance, I feel very disappointed that I was not awake for the birth, and that my partner was not with me.*'

'*With having a general I feel I missed out on the first moments.*'

One woman summed up her feelings very succinctly: '*One hour recovering from anaesthetic. Precious moments lost forever.*'

The overwhelming majority of women who commented on the type of anaesthetic used were pleased to be awake during the birth. For example, women who had been given spinal blocks were, on the whole, particularly content:

'I found the caesarean section to be less of an ordeal than I'd anticipated. It avoided a long, hard labour which may have ended as a section in any case. Spinal anaesthesia has the beauty of both worlds in that you avoid labour pains and are fully alert during the operation.'

'Listening to some other mothers who gave birth naturally I think I was lucky to have a spinal section with no pain and it was all over in one hour.'

For many women the two main advantages of being awake during a caesarean were, first, that they could be aware of the birth of their babies, seeing them and even holding them immediately, and second, being able to have their partner/friend with them during the operation. *'I found the spinal block operation fascinating and was awake to see the baby delivered immediately. It was also nice to know that my husband was there to see the birth and that I was able to talk to him right through the operation.'*

Epidurals were equally praised:

'I was very pleased with the epidural and the fact that this was an elective section. I would opt for this method in future rather than a general anaesthetic which I found extremely painful afterwards.'

'Having had an epidural anaesthesia I would recommend it. I think it should be available to all mothers, after-effects are minimal and ambulation I found much easier.'

'If I could have any more children I would not hesitate to have an epidural anaesthetic for a caesarean section. It was not as uncomfortable an operation as first thought.'

'The epidural was absolutely brilliant because I could feel him being born so felt I had participated. It was wonderful to be able to have my husband with me in theatre and to be talked through the whole thing – wouldn't have missed it for anything.'

The strength of opinion on this matter was at its highest from the women who after previous caesareans experienced an elective one. Many of these women had been given general anaesthesia the first time and so were in the best position to comment on the relative benefits of being awake or asleep. Their feelings were appropriately summed up by one woman: '*Obviously any woman would prefer a normal delivery but an elective section using a spinal or epidural anaesthetic is the next best thing. A caesarean birth can be a very positive and moving experience and with post-operative pain relief can easily be coped with.*'

Another woman commented on the relative after-effects of the different types of anaesthetic: '*I have had two types of caesarean anaesthetic, general and spinal. I must say with the spinal the after-effects are a lot easier to deal with due to the fact that you are more alert and there are less side effects.*'

One woman put her different experiences down to the length of time between her first and second operations and improvements in service that she believed had occurred in that time. '*My first caesarean was in 1981 after a long labour which did not progress and was done under general. Things have improved greatly in ten years and being awake this time made all the difference.*'

Obviously the women in the elective caesarean group were more likely to be prepared for the experience and to be in a situation to choose to be awake. These women appeared to have had much more satisfying experiences of caesarean section:

'*This is the second time by caesarean. The first was by general anaesthetic. Last time I felt cheated that I missed so much and did not see my baby properly until the next day. This time by spinal block was wonderful, we both saw him straight away and did not miss anything.*'

'*Everyone was very helpful, telling me what was going on. I felt very secure about being awake. It was a lot easier after the baby was born. Epidurals are a lot better than a general as you don't seem to be in much pain. My partner was able to be there which is a very good thing as they also know what's happening. The one big plus about epidurals is that you see your baby straight away which for me was the most emotional thing that I have ever encountered.*'

'*After having my first baby by emergency caesarean section under general anaesthetic I felt depressed and upset as I felt I had missed out a lot by not being awake during the birth. This time I had a much more pleasurable experience due to the fact that I was awake to see what was going on, I was able to see my baby straight after he was born and my husband was allowed in this time.*'

'*I much preferred the caesarean section by spinal anaesthetic as I was able to hold the baby immediately and the after-effects of the anaesthetic were minimal.*'

In part the after-effects of general anaesthesia appear to be more severe and debilitating than either epidural or spinal block anaesthesia, but the main advantage to mothers about being awake is that they are able to see their babies as soon as they are born.

'It's much better if you stay awake, there's no more pain and you get to see your baby straight away.'

'I am pleased that I was able to have this operation under epidural rather than a general anaesthetic. Thus allowing me to see the baby earlier and be part of the birth process.'

A few women expressed their regret at not being awake for their first caesareans in the light of their experiences with the second:

'When I had my first caesarean I was frightened to be awake but now that I know what it was like being awake with the second, I would have loved to have been awake the first time. It was a great feeling seeing the baby straight away.'

'I found the epidural better as you can see baby straight away. The first time I lost that bond with the baby, I didn't feel he was mine.'

Obviously each pregnancy and delivery must be judged according to its own specific circumstances and conditions but, given the evidence presented here, it must surely raise the question of whether it ought to be routine practice for the women to be awake in all possible cases when undergoing caesarean section. Another important point raised by this study is the need to prepare for caesarean birth early in pregnancy, if at all possible. This is better for the woman both physically and mentally and must surely be better for the hospital staff as well as the woman's partner. This point is highlighted in the words of one respondent:

'A caesarean section was queried throughout my pregnancy. An X-ray of my pelvis was taken as it is small. I feel I should have had a planned section and if I had I would have had an epidural. Instead I was made to go through full labour and then rushed to theatre for a section. My husband and I feel that we have both missed out on the birth of our son.'

However, it is rare today in the United Kingdom for it to be quite certain that a woman will need a caesarean, even where feto-pelvic disproportion is suspected. The good results achieved by midwives confirm that few healthy women in fact need caesareans.[2] As is shown in Chapter

---

2 Durrand, 1992.

8, there is great divergence of opinion among British consultants as to the indications for caesareans and there are some women who would prefer an elective caesarean rather than risk the possibility of an emergency operation. Therefore if a caesarean is needed, regional rather than general anaesthesia should be given and the partner should be present in theatre whether or not the woman is awake. This can contribute to the experience being as positive a one as possible and, if the woman can be awake, will enable her to see her baby as soon as it is born.

PARTNER'S ATTENDANCE AT A CAESAREAN

Women were asked: 'Did you have a friend/partner present for the birth?' (Table A2, page 180). The results demonstrated that just over half (55 per cent) of the women in the sample had their friend/partner present during the delivery. More of the women in the elective category had their partner/friend present during the operation – two out of three (65.9 per cent) – whereas less than half (46.3 per cent) of women having emergency operations were accompanied.

Women who did not have a partner present were asked why not. There were 102 answers given by the women in this category. The overwhelming majority of the explanations (79.4 per cent) were to do with hospital/doctor policy regarding caesarean sections or the fact that the emergency situation of the operation meant that either partners were not allowed in the operating theatre or they could not have got there on time even if they were allowed in.

Typical comments were as follows:

'Doctor didn't approve of husbands being present.'

'We were never offered the chance due to general anaesthetic.'

'He was not allowed to attend due to general anaesthetic.'

However, in a fifth of cases one or other of the couple had not wished attendance. One in seven (13.7 per cent) reasons related to the partner themselves: for example, they were too scared/nervous, they could not get time off work or they were unwell. The women said:

'He didn't feel he could have coped.'

'My partner was too scared.'

'My husband is squeamish.'

'My husband couldn't get time off work and therefore could not be at the birth.'

The final 6.9 per cent of reasons were that the woman did not want her friend/partner to be present. One woman stated that the reason her partner was not with her during the birth was that '*I didn't want anyone there.*'

The results indicate that the vast majority of women (93 per cent) would prefer to have a friend/partner with them during the birth and it is the organisation of hospital services which sometimes prevents this. If the main reason for not allowing a partner into the operating theatre is that the woman is asleep under general anaesthetic, this is an indication that women should be given epidural or spinal block anaesthetic wherever possible. However, there is no reason that the partner should not be present. Obstetricians are now used to this idea, but many anaesthetists need to be made aware of the importance to the couple that at least one partner is able to see the birth.

INFORMATION GIVEN TO WOMEN
Before the operation

Women were asked: 'Before the operation were you able to find out all you wanted to know about your condition and that of your nearly born baby?'

The results showed (Table A3, page 181) that a substantial majority (87.8 per cent) of the respondents felt that they had been kept adequately informed of their own and their baby's conditions. However, a discrepancy was found on this issue between the women who had had emergency operations and those having elective caesareans. Over one in six (18.2 per cent) of the women receiving emergency caesareans said that they were not able to find out all they wanted to know, compared with less than one in twenty (4.6 per cent) in the elective caesarean group. This is probably because in the emergency situation there is not enough time to inform women adequately of all that is happening. As one respondent commented: '*I knew nothing about a caesarean birth and there wasn't enough time to explain the procedure.*'

It appears that much of the dissatisfaction among the emergency caesarean group stemmed from their lack of preparation for an operative delivery. This raises questions about appropriate preparation for the potential of caesarean birth during the antenatal period, given that statistically one in eight women is likely to have a caesarean.

Information about treatment

Women were then asked: 'Were you kept informed of the treatment you were being given?' The overwhelming response was positive and 95.7 per cent answered 'yes' to this question.

Of the women who were not kept informed, one said she did not know *'how the pain killing treatments would have affected me'.*

Information about the baby's condition

The next question was: 'Do you feel that you were kept fully informed about your baby's condition?' The vast majority (91.7 per cent) answered this question affirmatively. Out of the seventeen women who gave a negative response, twelve (70.6 per cent) had an emergency caesarean, when there may not have been much time to communicate. Most of these women felt that they would have liked more information about their baby's condition. One woman said that she would have liked to have been told about the effects of the operation on her baby, for example the after-effects such as shock, anaemia and jaundice. Another said that she would have liked to have been told what risks the operation would have for her baby. Other comments related to the general condition of the baby before, during and immediately after the operation. One woman stated that her baby's condition was never discussed.

It was not the case, however, that all the women wanted more information. For example, one mother said: *'I was glad not to be told the full details until the next day.'* Similarly, another implied that more information would have made her feel worse: *'I was upset and it would have bothered me more if I knew baby was distressed.'*

Another mother expressed feelings of wanting to know more but also accepted that such information may have had a negative effect on her. She said: *'I would like to have been told about the baby's position in the womb, but perhaps this would have been disheartening.'*

It appears from these results that women were satisfied overall with the amount of information they received from the hospital staff. Among those who said that they were not kept fully informed, there were some women who did not necessarily want to know more.

Information about subsequent births

The women were asked: 'Have you been told what kind of birth to expect with your next pregnancy?' Of the 279 mothers who answered this question, just over half (51.6 per cent) had not been told. There appears to be great divergence between hospitals in terms of whether or not women are given information regarding what type of birth they should expect with subsequent pregnancies. Six out of the nine hospitals taking part in this study tended to give women this information.

Of the 135 women who were told what to expect, over half (57 per cent) were told that they would probably need another caesarean. Not surprisingly, almost three in five of these women (59.7 per cent) had had previous caesareans. This advice appeared to be fairly consistent among the different hospitals.

The respondents were then asked: 'How do you feel about this? (e.g. frightened/pleased/sad/mixed/other)' Of the women who were told that they would probably need another caesarean for any subsequent pregnancies, almost two in five (38.9 per cent) said that they had 'mixed feelings' about it. One in seven (13.9 per cent) were 'pleased' with this advice. One in nine (11.1 per cent) reported negative feelings such as 'frightened', 'sad', 'disappointed' and 'apprehensive'. For women who had been told that they would be able to deliver normally in the future, two in five (40 per cent) said that they were 'pleased' about it and a further 10 per cent reported other positive feelings such as 'fine' and 'relieved'. One in ten (10 per cent) had 'mixed' feelings about it. Only one woman in the sample said that she felt 'frightened' about this prospect.

Women's understanding at the time of birth

The mothers were asked: 'At the time did you understand why a caesarean section was needed?', to which 276 mothers assented and therefore 92 per cent understood why their caesarean was needed. Only 9 women (3 per cent) answered 'no' to this question. The remaining respondents said that they did not know or could not remember.

DO WOMEN WHO HAVE CAESAREANS SUFFER?

Women were asked: 'Do you consider that you suffered as a result of having a caesarean?' The results (Table A4, page 181) showed that three in five women overall (60.1 per cent) said that they did not feel that they had suffered from the operation. However, some difference was found between women giving birth by elective sections and those having emergency operations. Four out of five (80 per cent) of the women having elective operations said they did not feel that they had suffered, compared to just over half (55.9 per cent) of the women receiving emergency caesareans. Comments from women as to why they felt they had suffered can be analysed as follows.

Suffering caused by the pain of the operation

The overwhelming majority of comments related to the pain, although it seems that the level varies according to each woman's own physiological response, the skill of the obstetrician who performed the caesarean and the effectiveness of the post-operative pain relief. Two typical quotes were the following:

'I would much prefer a normal birth as the pain you have is over. But with caesarean you seem to have quite a bit of pain and discomfort for quite a while after. Also it takes you a lot longer to get back to normal which I shall find very hard.'

'I had a 14 hour labour and have at this stage endured a further week of pain and discomfort. I cannot sit down or stand with the baby in my arms, I have to have him reached to me and it's very frustrating.'

Women who had experienced previous vaginal deliveries felt the pain of caesarean section particularly worthy of comment:

'Much less enjoyable and more painful than a natural birth.'

'My natural labour was less painful.'

One respondent who had experienced a previous caesarean found that the second operation was not as painful afterwards as the first, which may relate to her being better prepared and knowing what to expect. *'The first section was very painful and I was shocked at the severity of it. For the second one I was a bit wary because I knew of the pain I was in with the first. But it was nowhere near as bad.'*

Many women felt that the post-operative pain adversely affected their ability to cope with their newborn babies. One woman said that she had suffered *'because of not being able to see my baby properly as I was very sore and couldn't manoeuvre the same'*.

Some people believe that the caesarean is a painless way of giving birth and that women who have caesareans have somehow taken the 'soft' option in not having to suffer labour pains. The fact that the mothers have undergone major abdominal surgery and have a high degree of post-operative pain may not always be fully realised by other women in the hospital. Two mothers made statements to this effect:

'It is annoying that other Mums think you've had an easy time without the labour. They do not realise it is really hard getting yourself pulled together afterwards.'

'Myself and other women who have had babies by caesareans feel very annoyed when people who had normal deliveries think we were lucky and had an "easy way out" as recovery is very long and painful. It is many months before you feel well again.'

Differences emerged in the experience of pain between women having elective operations and those having emergency caesareans. Almost one out of three (32.3 per cent) women having emergency operations felt more pain than they had expected, compared to only one in five (21.2 per cent) of women having elective sections.

Suffering caused by not being able to give birth naturally

Many women felt a severe sense of loss at not being able to give birth naturally. One woman from the elective caesarean group said that she felt that she had suffered *'emotionally because I wanted to do it naturally by myself with little pain relief.'* Another said: *'I had no worries about giving birth by caesarean but I am sad that I cannot have a normal birth.'*

Comments from the emergency caesarean group included: *'You can't class caesarean as giving birth, I don't feel as if I have really had a baby.'* Another felt that she had *'lost out on being able to deliver normally'*.

Even when understanding the necessity for the operation in their own case, some women still felt a severe sense of loss:

'It felt safer for me and baby at the time, although I am still upset that I was not able to see natural birth through.'

'I would have liked to have a normal delivery. However caesarean was a life-saving operation for both myself and baby.'

Suffering caused by the effects on 'bonding'

Many respondents in the survey felt that being separated from their babies immediately after the birth had a deleterious effect on their ability to bond appropriately. This was particularly true for the women who had experienced emergency caesareans, partly because this group of mothers was more likely to have been given general anaesthesia. Furthermore they were more likely to have given birth to babies who needed specialist treatment following the birth. However, it must be remembered that some mothers who have delivered vaginally find that they are unable to spend time with their baby after birth because either they or their babies need urgent treatment. Some other mothers have had a normal delivery and spent time holding their baby after birth but find that they do not form the special attachment to their baby until hours, days or even weeks later. Forming a relationship with a new baby is a unique process which every parent experiences in their own way.

Typical comments from the survey were as follows:

'The initial bonding feelings between Mum and baby seem to have taken longer to take place.'

'I feel that caesarean takes away the vital importance of the bonding between mother and baby in the first two days.'

Many women accepted the necessity for the operation but were still concerned about the effects on their bonding with their baby. *'I feel it was necessary for the health of my baby, but I feel I missed those precious first moments of life. I also feel that having a caesarean limits the care you can give your baby.'*

The experience of one respondent sums up the feelings of many regarding those first important minutes after the birth:

'The first caesarean I had was in '86. After 12 hours I had only dilated 3 cm. I had a general anaesthetic which meant I didn't see my baby and needed my visitors to tell me what she looked like. I was very upset by this so they brought me her to look at during the night. It took me a few months to form a loving bond. This time I feel very different. As I saw baby immediately the bond has been there from the first moment.'

Over half the women in this sample saw their baby as soon as it was born. More than three in five (66.2 per cent) of the mothers having elective caesareans saw their babies immediately; less than two in five (39.4 per cent) of the emergency caesarean group did so. This corresponds with the number of women who had epidural and general anaesthesia.

Suffering caused by the lengthy recovery period Many of the women commented on the lengthy recovery period and the fact that they were not able to be up and about with their baby soon after the operation.

'I am satisfied my caesareans were necessary for the safety of the babies in both instances. However, it must surely be the worst way to give birth as just when you need to be fit to cope with a new baby, you are coping with a major operation. I found it terribly frustrating.'

'I feel relieved that such intervention is possible as it does obviously save the lives of newborn babies. However it is upsetting when for the first days or so you have to rely on the midwives and other staff so much for the care of your newborn.'

Suffering in general   A recurring theme on the question of how women
────────────────── felt they had suffered because of the caesarean
section points to women not being adequately prepared mentally for an
operative delivery. '*After a trouble-free pregnancy it is difficult to accept
being an "invalid" and dependent on others.*'

Similarly we can see how the long recovery period following the caesarean has an adverse effect on women, especially when they have other
children to think about. '*I had hoped to recover from this birth much
more quickly than last time, whereas now presumably it will be as before,
but harder, thanks to a two-year-old!*'

Some women expressed relief at not having to do all the caring for
the baby in the first day or so and were pleased to have the hospital
staff on hand to help out. One woman said that she felt '*Okay at time,
but very sore afterwards, although I miss not having baby with me.
Don't know how I would have coped if they had given me baby the
next day, I was very weak and tired.*'

Other general comments that women made regarding how they felt
they had suffered centred around conditions caused to their baby because
of the operation, for example problems with breathing, and general
discomfort caused to themselves in terms of headaches, wind, depression
and permanent scarring to the body.

Other results showed that four out of five (84 per cent) women having
caesareans felt tired after the operation, and over half (55.3 per cent)
felt weak. To a lesser extent women felt sick and/or depressed, one in
six (17.3 per cent) and one in seven (15 per cent) respectively. However,
women who had had emergency operations reported all of these feelings
more than the women who had had elective caesareans. The most startling difference was in the case of depression. Over twice as many emergency caesarean women reported feeling this post-operatively, almost
one in five (19.6 per cent), compared to one in eleven (9.1 per cent) of
the women who had had elective caesareans. Of course, one cannot
overlook the effect that general anaesthesia may have on women's emotional states, but this finding may, once again, indicate a lack of preparation for operative delivery among women and raise questions about
the need for more antenatal information.

CAESAREANS AS A POSITIVE EXPERIENCE

Although many women in this study
concentrated on the negative aspects
of operative birth and some sug-
gested ways in which things could be improved for caesarean patients,
it is important to point out that many women were extremely happy to

have had caesarean sections, either because of their gratitude in terms of a successful outcome for their babies or alternatively because they enjoyed the whole experience and found it to be a rewarding one. Many women emphasised their gratitude that the operation was available to help them out of what they perceived to be a very difficult situation. One woman explained how she felt after the operation: *'Painful after-wards, unable to care for baby and my other children as well as I had hoped for. Complications of wound infection are a setback. But thank goodness caesarean sections are available when one cannot deliver vaginally.'*

Others stressed the advantages of caesarean birth in terms of the outcome for their babies:

'If a caesarean was not done my daughter would never have been born normally, except at huge risk to her and myself.'

'It was unavoidable and in the best interests of the baby. Whilst it will take a while to recover it is comforting to know the baby is now safe and well.'

One woman said that she was not upset at having to have a caesarean even though she would have preferred not to: *'I had previously been given the option of caesarean section and decided against it. However, I do not regret having had a section (except for the discomfort I'm feeling) and do not feel cheated of a vaginal delivery.'*

Another expressed her surprise that the operation was not as bad as she had expected: *'I was very reluctant to have a caesarean but decided towards the end of a 16 hour labour it was the sensible option. There is some discomfort but I probably would have got that anyway with a normal delivery. I am very pleased with the size and position of scar, it is really different to what I expected.'*

For many women the outcome justified the means:

'As soon as they said you will have to have a section, I became very upset and cried a lot, even though I thoroughly understood the circum-stances and knew it was for the very best for my baby and me. But as soon as I came round and saw my husband with my beautiful son I was glad it was all over and glad I had a section. I DON'T REGRET IT ONE BIT AND NEITHER DOES MY HUSBAND.' (emphasis in original)

Many women found the whole experience very rewarding. For some it was because they felt they had been given a reasonable trial of labour before the operation, and for others it was because they were awake during it and were therefore able to feel that they had taken part in the process and seen their babies as they were born. One woman who was awake for the operation said: *'I was very impressed by what a beautiful experience a caesarean could be. I think I would have been more disappointed if I had not been allowed such a full trial of labour but having experienced this the caesarean was a very enjoyable climax to the labour.'*

WOMEN'S ADVICE TO OTHER WOMEN

Some women in the study, acknowledging the general feeling of failure among caesarean patients, offered words of advice and support to those who are to follow them onto the operating table. One woman was reassuring about the bond she felt with her baby: *'I think that many women feel as though they have failed if they have to give birth by caesarean. But I definitely don't find this to be true as the love you have for your baby is just as strong with a caesarean as with a vaginal birth.'*

Another respondent offered very practical advice:

'1. Don't try and do too much too soon in hospital. You've to be easy on yourself so you can do more later (remember that you've had a major operation).
2. Physically once you're up and walking keep your back straight.
3. Allow yourself a good cry when you want one.'

CAESAREAN SECTIONS AND BREASTFEEDING

Mothers were asked: 'Did you want to breastfeed your baby?' The results revealed that over half (51.9 per cent) of the women having caesarean sections said that they wanted to breastfeed. Over two in five (41.9 per cent) of the women in this sample said that they did not want to breastfeed. This compares with national figures of 63 per cent of women giving birth in Britain who chose to breastfeed in 1990, 64 per cent in England and Wales, and 50 per cent in Scotland.[3]

Those women who did not want to breastfeed were asked about their decision. The majority (73 per cent) said that their decision not to breastfeed stemmed from their being 'not too keen on breast-feeding'. This may indicate the need for more positive information for women about breastfeeding. Of these women, 11.5 per cent said that they had 'changed their mind' about breastfeeding and a similar number (13.1 per cent) said that they did not want to breastfeed their baby because they 'felt too ill'.

....

3 Office of Population Censuses and Surveys, 1992.

Less common reasons given by women for not wanting to breastfeed were that they 'had no milk', had 'inverted nipples' or because the 'baby wouldn't take to breastfeeding'. But these reasons are widespread among all women who begin to breastfeed their babies and then give up,[4] and are generally the result of inadequate professional support for breastfeeding.[5] Some women felt that breastfeeding was inconvenient so they wanted to share the responsibility for feeding, or they preferred bottle feeding. However, once a woman has learned how to breastfeed, she may find it more convenient than bottle feeding because there are no bottles to make up and there is no formula to buy. Other reasons related to previous experiences such as failure with breastfeeding and suffering from breast abscesses which can also be the result of poor professional support and a lack of correct information. One woman from each group said that they were 'too sore' (usually the result of poor positioning of the baby at the breast) and two women from the emergency caesarean group said that they could not breastfeed because their babies were in the special care baby unit.

According to the Infant Feeding 1990 survey, having a caesarean delivery under general anaesthetic or having a low birthweight baby were both associated with early cessation of breastfeeding. However, mothers whose babies received special care were no more likely to stop breastfeeding in the first two weeks than other mothers.[6] Women's decisions as to whether to breastfeed and whether to continue breastfeeding are very complex and influenced by many deep-seated factors such as culture, the practice of their peer group and the attitude of their partner and other members of their family. When women have had a caesarean birth, the post-operative pain and the possible feelings of inadequacy from having not given birth vaginally can be added to these influences. For some women, succeeding at breastfeeding is even more important because they have not had a normal birth.

The results of our survey showed that it was the women who had emergency caesareans who were more likely to have been given general anaesthesia and who felt that this had a deleterious effect on their experience of childbirth. It is therefore possible to deduce that general anaesthesia and the accompanying feelings of illness may have had an effect on women's decisions on whether or not to breastfeed their babies. Even women who tried to breastfeed had problems and these may have led

....
4 Office of Population Censuses and Surveys, 1992.
5 Royal College of Midwives, 1991.
6 Office of Population Censuses and Surveys, 1992, pp. 40–5.

them to stop breastfeeding because of inadequate professional support.

As breastfeeding is better for all babies, there are therefore serious implications for the babies of women who have emergency caesareans under general anaesthetic. There needs to be recognition that women who have had caesareans have an increased need for support for breastfeeding, both practical and emotional. This is corroborated by the *Successful Breastfeeding* handbook for midwives, which states: 'There is no evidence to support the long-established belief that caesarean section itself has any deleterious effect on the establishment of lactation. The mother will probably require more help to find a comfortable feeding position and with attaching the baby to the breast in the first few days then she would if she had been vaginally delivered'.[7]

CAESAREAN SECTION – THE WOMEN SPEAK

From the results of this survey and the responses of women to caesarean sections it can be seen that mothers generally have a much better experience of operative delivery if they are adequately prepared for it and are supported by staff in terms of being kept informed throughout the whole process. This point is borne out by the fact that women having elective caesareans report greater satisfaction with the operation than those who have had emergency sections.

'*It was a wonderful experience. Because it was elective we were able to organise for the birth, my partner was present and prepared well. He was able to organise leave to be with us, this would have been difficult under less certain circumstances.*'

'*Being an elective section I found I was much better prepared physically and mentally than my first section. Recovery from an elective section was speedier and not as traumatic to both myself and baby.*'

'*Having had three sections, the first being emergency by general anaesthetic, not very pleasant, second and third spinal and a great experience. I think all the information and advice you can be given by the staff helps immensely with both the operation and what the after-effects will be. This being so, there would be no great shocks. I was given brilliant advice and care, so all my experiences have been very good.*'

One woman explained how simply knowing that she might need another caesarean made it easier to cope: '*With the first caesarean there was great disappointment and feeling that I had suffered a labour for*

---

7 Royal College of Midwives, 1991, p. 77.

nothing. This time I was fairly optimistic about delivering normally but knew there was the possibility of a second caesarean. Therefore I don't feel so let down this time.'

Some respondents were aware that they might have felt better if they had been better prepared for the possibility of caesarean birth.

'I wished it could be explained about a caesarean birth earlier in pregnancy.'

'It would have been better if I was more prepared for it.'

One woman described how her lack of knowledge about caesareans made the experience worse for her: *'Caesareans should be termed as normal operations not minor operations. All along I thought a caesarean wasn't a big deal. I was told how it is done but not how you feel afterwards.'* (This woman made specific reference to the amount of pain encountered after the operation.)

WOMEN'S ADVICE TO HOSPITAL STAFF

Some women felt able to advise medical practitioners on the use of caesareans, for example saying that it should only be used when all other options have been exhausted. One woman said that *'It is best used only in emergency cases.'* Another stated: *'Emergency section decisions should be made as early as possible as a long period in labour beforehand is very traumatic.'* These two comments exemplify the significant divergence of opinion between women on whether caesareans should only be used as a last resort, when the woman has been given every chance to deliver vaginally. It is clear from the survey that some women wish to be allowed to labour for as long as possible whereas others would prefer a caesarean to be recommended earlier to give them time to come to terms with it. The only solution is for hospital staff to get to know each woman individually, to maintain good communication in labour and to invite her to join in any decisions made about her care.

One woman gave very specific advice:

'1. It should be a last resort.
2. More information should be impressed on expectant mothers – so that they appreciate that it could happen to them.'

This second point highlights the feelings of many women about lack of information given to expectant women. The question of what is taught at antenatal classes was a recurring theme:

'I think that much more should be taught about caesareans at ante-natal

classes to prepare women for the after-effects as it seems commonplace nowadays.'

'I would have liked to know more ante-natally about different kinds of pain relief given post-caesarean section. It might be helpful to consider each case individually and not just prescribe routine painkillers. Otherwise I was impressed by the standard of care and information given to me.'

Many women felt that improvements in post-operative care could be made:

'I think that caesarean patients should really be given more rest and not expected to be up and around within 24 hours to be looking after baby. I felt that for the first 3 days that the baby could have been took off me at night, and bottle fed, and then left with me when she was quiet in the day and breast fed. But the second day I was up, and doing nearly everything by the third day, which caused me stress because I couldn't quite manage because of the pain I was in. It left me feeling inadequate as a mother, and I wanted to do more.'

'The most important thing for recovery afterwards is sleep and you don't get any on a post-natal ward with up to 10 other mums and babies. Caesarean patients should have their own rooms/side wards for recovery as I did after my first one.'

'I feel support for caesarean mothers is more important once they are home as depression is not always immediate and affected me several months after my previous caesarean sections.'

THE ATTITUDE OF THE HOSPITAL STAFF

One of the most important factors affecting whether or not women had a positive experience of caesarean section, besides being fully informed and being awake during the operation, was the attitude of the hospital staff. Not surprisingly, those women who were helped through the experience by caring and supportive staff had a much better experience overall. One woman commented on the attitude of staff on the way to the operating theatre: *'The atmosphere was very relaxed when they took me up to theatre, even managed to get me laughing. My husband and I found this a great help.'*

For those women who were awake during the operation the attitude of the theatre staff was equally important.

'I felt frightened but confident at the same time. The theatre staff made

me feel very special, I had lots of attention. I was overwhelmed with gratitude when they delivered our baby.'

'The third section was the best of the lot, much more straightforward – and went according to plan. The theatre staff were a tremendous help talking me through the operation. After, I felt on top of the world and very relaxed.'

'The staff were very supportive and were always reassuring me throughout the whole birth because it was my first birth and having a hard time as well. If I have to have a caesarean again I would hope that I would be fortunate enough to have similar staff as I had for my first.'

'I found the staff in the theatre very helpful and friendly which was very satisfying and made things a lot easier.'

One woman pointed out how a friendly atmosphere in the theatre helps the woman and does not interfere with efficiency: *'The relaxed atmosphere of the theatre was good and should be encouraged. It did not at any time seem to interfere with its smooth and efficient running.'*

Of course support and understanding on the part of hospital staff is equally important post-operatively. *'I felt quite happy about this last section. The operation went fine and I have felt very well through the recovery stage. I have received very good support from the staff and this I feel is most important. They have given me the help when I have asked and have let me do things in my own time.'*

One woman commented on how the attitude of the staff helped her get over the shock of having to have an emergency section: *'An emergency section is very frightening because you are not prepared for it. But if the hospital you are in has good and caring staff where nothing is too much, makes the difference on your outlook of things.'*

Clearly the attitude and outlook of staff interacts with other factors such as being adequately informed and, preferably, being awake during the operation, to enable caesarean patients to have a positive experience. These thoughts are appropriately summed up in the words of one of the respondents:

'Two years ago I had a "semi-emergency" section under general anaesthetic in a different hospital. I was not offered an epidural and even had I had one my husband would not have been allowed to stay with me. So bad did I feel the experience and recovery to have been that I changed to a hospital 20 miles further away to avoid a repetition. Although the outcome was essentially the same, i.e. caesarean, the experience was

completely different – everyone seemed to be "on my side" this time. I was quite happy about the ultimate decision, hence I feel I am recovering much better. I think the two crucial factors in this are:
i) the attitude of the staff on the labour ward, and
ii) epidural anaesthesia, which enabled both me and my husband to be present for the birth.'

SUMMING UP WOMEN'S COMMENTS

One of the most important findings of this study is that women who are awake for their caesareans tend to have much better experiences of the operation and report less suffering. There are a number of other reasons that it is preferable for women to be awake for the operation:

1. The women are conscious of all that is happening and therefore feel that they have participated in the birth.
2. The mothers are able to see their babies as soon as they are born.
3. Their partners are able to be present at the birth and to play a role.
4. The women do not have to cope with the after-effects of a general anaesthetic.

This raises the important question of whether it ought to be routine practice for women to be awake for caesarean sections in all possible cases. In these 300 deliveries by caesarean, only two in five (39.7 per cent) were performed with the woman awake. Even in the case of elective operations, only three out of five caesareans were done with the woman awake. This is the result of hospital or consultant policy rather than women's preference, as comments from women overwhelmingly suggest that they would rather be awake.

One of the most startling observations to come out of this research is the fact that many women are relatively unprepared for operative delivery. Caesarean birth is mentioned at antenatal classes but not all women attend these classes and the philosophy of 'it'll never happen to me' may come into play, in particular when the pregnancy has been normal.

It also points to the fact that there is a lack of understanding generally about caesarean birth. Some women see it as a 'soft' option and do not realise the pain, discomfort, lack of mobility and lengthy recovery that it entails. Medical practitioners do not always realise that women who are better informed often have better experiences of operative birth. Obviously this is not always possible in an emergency situation but does indicate that all pregnant women need to have full knowledge of caesarean section, whether they are seen to be 'at risk' in terms of possibly needing a section or not. Similarly hospital staff need to be sensitive to the post-operative needs and feelings of women who have had caesareans as they will not always be able to deal with their newborns as well as they had expected and this can cause stress and depression.

From the comments made by the women in the survey it is clear that many experience very mixed feelings about the operation. Obviously they are thankful that it is available and understand the necessity in certain circumstances. Yet because the majority of women are incapacitated by the surgery, they are unable to fulfil what they perceive to be their full maternal role with their babies. This will inevitably lead to conflict for the women concerned.

It appears that, on the whole, women are kept informed about their condition and that of their baby. However, information is often lacking in terms of the procedure for caesarean section and the effects on women post-operatively. If women are to make informed decisions and to be empowered to take a full and rewarding part in the birth of their children, they need to realise that caesarean birth is a possibility and to be given appropriate information in order to reduce feelings of shock, disappointment and resentment. In particular women should be made aware of the relative advantages and disadvantages of the different types of anaesthesia used for caesarean operations, the possibility that they may not see their baby immediately after birth and how they are likely to feel post-operatively. It should be explained that there will be reduced mobility and some pain.

At the same time, it needs to be said that in most cases where an emergency caesarean is necessary, there is time not only for the choice and administration of local anaesthesia but also for giving all information relevant to the woman. It is only in the case of a real emergency, perhaps if the woman is bleeding heavily or having fits, that this is not the case. Also, women need to have an accurate idea of the real chances of having a caesarean. Although the overall rate for caesareans is one in eight, of women who go into labour normally it is about one in twenty-five; and for women who have had one normal birth, the rate is even lower, at one in fifty.

CHAPTER EIGHT

POLICIES OF BRITISH CONSULTANTS

*Our caesarean rate has gone up 300 percent in the
fifteen years since I have been here and yet the salvage of
small babies has not changed one jot. The reason that
the caesarean section rate is going up is that we are
all scared stiff of litigation.*

WE have seen that the debate over whether the caesarean rate is too high
has proceeded through this century. In fact it was in 1949 that G. W.
Theobold told the *BMJ* that he had a dream in which 'All deliveries were
by caesarean, to facilitate which a zip fastener has been invented'.[1]

In order to find out more recent thoughts on the subject, we took a
random sample of over 400 consultant obstetricians in England and Wales
and included at least one doctor in every hospital as well as all Scottish
obstetric consultants. We have published our results in the *British Journal
of Obstetrics and Gynaecology* and have included more details about the
methodology in Appendix B.[2] The analysis we provide here is both fuller
and made to be much more relevant to parents. It also contains data from
our fourth mailing in 1992 which brought our response rate in England and
Wales up to 70 per cent: a total of 352 consultants.

The chapter is in three sections. In the first part we consider the attitudes
of consultants to performing caesareans in different circumstances and their
reasons for the number performed. In the second part we discuss the care
of the pregnant woman and the consultants' attitude to whether she should
be awake or asleep for the operation and whether her partner should be able
to attend the caesarean birth. Finally, we draw some general conclusions.

REASONS FOR DOING A CAESAREAN
Use of caesarean early in pregnancy to save a baby

With the improved level of postnatal care
some obstetricians feel it worthwhile to
carry out a caesarean on distressed
fetuses before term. In order to find out
their exact views, there were two linked

---

1 Theobold, 1949, p. 147.
2 Savage and Francome, 1993.

questions which can be analysed together. The first was: 'Would you perform a CS to deliver a woman at 24 weeks gestation for fetal distress?' The second asked: 'Would you perform a CS to deliver a woman at 26 weeks gestation for fetal distress?' The results show (Table A5, page 181) that one-quarter of British consultants may perform a caesarean at twenty-four weeks for fetal distress. One consultant commented: 'At 23/52 I would not do a caesarean but after that there is a good chance of survival in our neonatal service.' One factor possibly concerning the consultants who would not perform a caesarean at twenty-four weeks is that the baby may have other problems, so that by performing a caesarean at this stage they may be delivering a baby which is handicapped and will not survive.

More typical was a consultant from Wales who said he would not carry out a caesarean at twenty-four weeks 'unless there were exceptional circumstances'. Another from the Yorkshire Region said she would carry out a caesarean at twenty-four weeks but made it a condition that 'fetal abnormality had been excluded previously'. On the question of a caesarean at twenty-four weeks, one answered 'depends' and further said that 'Other factors will influence but the tendency is NO at 24 weeks.' A doctor from the Trent Region said he would not carry out a caesarean at twenty-four weeks 'unless there was a catastrophic history of fetal wastage' (by this he meant that the woman had previous miscarriages or perinatal deaths). A doctor from the Northern Region said he would occasionally perform a caesarean at twenty-four weeks for fetal distress but that it would depend on various factors including parental attitude. A slightly different point was made by a consultant from the South Western Region who said he would not monitor the woman and so he would not be aware of any fetal distress. Others from different regions illustrated this point.

However, by twenty-six weeks consultants were much more positive towards carrying out a caesarean for fetal distress. At this stage three in ten (30.5 per cent) said that they would perform one, and over half replied that it would depend. Only one in seven (13.4 per cent) would not perform a caesarean in any circumstances at this gestation. One reason for the difference may be the size of the baby; a consultant from the Yorkshire Region said he would carry out a caesarean if the scan suggested that the fetus was 800 g or more. Another from the Wessex Region said he 'would now accept a birthweight estimate of 750 grams at 26 weeks.' A third from the Yorkshire Region took a positive line on the grounds that 50 per cent of the babies would survive at this stage.

Of the consultants who said that their decision would depend on the circumstances at twenty-six weeks, one commented that the decision would depend 'on parental understanding and other factors such as mother's age'. Another said he would do a caesarean at twenty-six weeks 'after clinical estimate and sonal investigation'. A third consultant who was from the Northern Region said he might carry out a caesarean 'depending on fetal condition and the state of the cervix'. One from the East Anglia Region said he would carry out a caesarean depending on 'All else being normal and if the outcome was expected to be good.'

An obstetrician from the Yorkshire Region said he would carry out a caesarean if the woman had lost a few previous pregnancies. Another from this region made a similar point that he would carry one out if the mother was older and there was a history of infertility. The age of the woman was a factor to which many consultants from most regions referred. One said he would do one 'only if it were a particularly precious pregnancy'.

A consultant from the Northern Region said she would consider 'Particular circumstances and availability of paediatric resources.' Another consultant from the north pointed out that there were problems with carrying out caesareans at twenty-six weeks because the intensive treatment unit was 100 miles away at Newcastle. Another consultant from the Yorkshire Region said he would carry out a caesarean 'if the special care baby unit had an available intensive care cot'. A second from this region said he would carry out a caesarean depending on the severity of distress and the 'work load in the Special Care Baby Unit'. Others also mentioned the need for the beds to be available in SCBU. Another from North West Thames commented that the decision 'depends on opinion of paediatricians. We would prefer transfer in utero if time permits (we cannot do long term ventilation on neonates).'

A consultant from the Yorkshire Region said his unit had no neonatal intensive care unit on site, so paediatric opinion would be sought. This viewpoint is similar to that of an East Anglian obstetrician who commented that the caesarean would depend on 'estimated prognosis and liaison with paediatricians for a decision'.

A consultant from the Trent Region said he was very unlikely to perform a caesarean at twenty-six weeks but it would depend on 'obstetric history and the certainty of dates'. Another from North West Thames said 'we keep a watch on neonatal survival figures which influence our decisions'.

A number of consultants pointed out that one factor which would influence their feelings was the cause of the fetal distress. One from the Trent Region made it clear that the decision to operate would only go ahead with complete parental support: 'If the background circumstances suggested that the fetus was likely to be healthier a caesarean would be *recommended*. However, the parents' wishes (after suitable counselling) would always be followed.'

Some of those who did not ever carry out caesareans at twenty-six weeks mentioned their lack of facilities. One from North West Thames said they did no caesareans at this stage: 'because we have no neonatal intensive care facilities we would make an in utero transfer to a regional centre if appropriate eg severe pre-eclampsia'. Another from North West Thames, in answer to the question about fetal distress at twenty-six weeks, said: 'Not at present, we've not an adequate special care baby unit.' Overall three quarters (76 per cent) of consultants reported that they had an SCBU.

Breech deliveries   There has been a great amount of debate about whether to perform a caesarean if the baby is breech (bottom first). In the early 1980s it was becoming routine to carry out a caesarean for breech in the United States and the percentage of breech presentations delivered by caesarean rose from 11.6 per cent in 1970 to 60.1 per cent in 1978.[3] This was despite the fact that New York City data showed no decline in mortality for breech babies over the period. The US government-appointed task force argued against always performing a caesarean for breech.[4] In Britain, too, the percentage of caesareans for breech has increased, and so in this study we asked the following question: 'Does your firm (team) have a policy of elective caesarean for breech presentation?' A total of 344 consultants answered this question. Of these 50 said they did have a policy of elective caesareans (14.5 per cent of the respondents); 178 doctors (52 per cent) said they did not have such a policy, and just over a third (106) said that it 'depends'.

These figures show that there is division within the British obstetric profession over this issue, so that in one in seven cases of breech presentation the woman in labour would have no option but a caesarean. However, the same woman with a different consultant in a different hospital would be given every opportunity to deliver vaginally.

Repeat caesarean   We asked the obstetricians: 'Do you adhere to the policy once a caesar, always a caesar?' The results (Table A6, page 181) show that only 1.1 per cent of consultants in

3 Carson and Francome, 1983, p. 6.
4 National Institutes of Health, 1982, p. 13.

England and Wales follow this dictum compared to 4.1 per cent in Scotland. This may be one factor leading to Scotland having a higher caesarean rate than England and Wales.

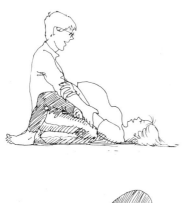

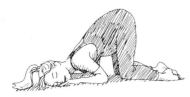

We felt that doctors might, however, differ a great deal in the proportion of women they allowed to deliver vaginally, and so we asked those who did not always do a caesarean: 'What proportion of women with previous caesareans had vaginal deliveries in the past year in your firm (team)?' The results showed that there was a wide difference in practice in England and Wales with 5.6 per cent of doctors achieving a vaginal delivery in over four out of five (80 per cent) women while 13.7 per cent proceeded to vaginal delivery in less than four cases out of ten (40 per cent). Few had accurate data and most gave us estimates.

One doctor from the Yorkshire region stated that the deliveries had to be divided into those with recurring and others with non-recurring indications. He suggested that in his practice 60 per cent of those with non-recurring indications followed a caesarean with a vaginal birth. We shall be considering the whole issue of vaginal birth after caesarean more fully in the next chapter.

Consultants' views about changes in their personal caesarean rate

Our respondents were asked about their experiences over the last five years. Two in five (39 per cent) reported little or no change, but of the other three-fifths the majority had an increase to report. The main reason mentioned was the fear of litigation. We shall see that this was a major reason in explaining the rise in caesarean births in Britain. However, a wide variety of reasons were discussed. A doctor from South East Thames, whose caesarean rate had increased over the five years from 11.6 to 15.8 per cent, said changes were related to 'critical assessment of post maturity and failed inductions'. Two consultants said that changes depended 'on the registrar's personality and experience'. Another commented that the increase was 'probably due to the inexperience of the junior staff'.

Several of those who reported increasing rates said that 'Registrars misread monitors.' Different reasons were proposed by a consultant from South East Thames, who said his rate had risen because of 'Patients' unwillingness to submit to another labour, also at risk pregnancy and litigation.' Thus two of the three reasons he gave for the increase were not related to improved health of the baby. A consultant from the South East Thames Region was one of those who said that safety was important and that his firm's caesarean rate had increased because of 'understanding that the procedure is very safe (as safe as SVD [spontaneous vertex delivery]) if done with epidural and electively.'

One commented on 'An awareness that couples have few children.' Thus some consultants were feeling the pressure that if there were problems, a caesarean might be the solution.

The evidence from individual consultants' practice can show wide swings. A good example came from the Northern Region. One firm's number of caesareans increased from 184 in 1986 to 238 in 1987 and then went back to 186 in 1988, with no substantial change in the number of deliveries. The consultant commented: 'the temporary increase in the middle years was due to the registrar's attitude'. This suggests that in 1987 some women had a caesarean that may have been unnecessary.

Of those doctors reporting a reduction in the rates, one from South West Thames said there was 'no obvious reason for the change but the rate has been going down'. Another commented on a reduction due to vaginal birth after caesarean and said there were 'increased attempts at trial of scar'. Of those who said the rate had reduced because of fewer failed inductions, one commented: 'The rate has reduced because of selection in induction policy.'

Reasons for the rise in the British caesarean rate In our survey we asked consultant obstetricians the following question: 'The British caesarean rate rose from 2.7% in 1958 to 11% in 1986. What would you say were the major reasons for the change during this period?' The results are provided in Table 8.1 below. The rise in Scotland is to a higher level and so we have separated the results obtained from north of the border.

The reasons the doctors gave can be divided into three groups. Over 40 per cent of the reasons were positive: doctors pointed out, for example, that caesareans are safer these days. However, some of the reasons were negative and in this group the largest single factor, mentioned by almost half the consultants, was litigation. Thus some doctors

Table 8.1   *Reasons for the rise in the British caesarean rate*

Reasons	England and Wales	Scotland	Total	% doctors
Positive				
Better care has improved fetal survival	59	13	72	22.0
Improved safety (inc. anaesthesia)	43	18	61	18.7
Increased expectations mothers/parents	30	7	37	11.3
To reduce perinatal morbidity	26	8	34	10.4
Better diagnosis of baby's problems	21	1	22	6.7
Better monitoring	17	4	21	6.4
Lower perinatal mortality rates	13	5	18	5.5
Abandonment of difficult forceps	10	4	14	4.3
Improved obstetric practice	10	3	13	4.0
Compassion for mothers	5	4	9	2.8
Increase for IUGR	4	3	7	2.1
Patient choice/request	6		6	1.8
Reduce risk of brain damage	3	2	5	1.5
Improved antenatal assessment	3		3	0.9
Other (benefits of CS)	4		4	1.2
Total	254	72	326	
Neutral				
Fetal monitoring	51	10	61	18.7
Breech (inc. a few management of malpresentation)	40	8	48	14.7
Long labour now not acceptable	11	9	20	6.1
Active management of labour	12	4	16	4.9
Repeat caesarean	8	0	8	2.4
Hospital deliveries	2	0	2	0.6
Twins	2	0	2	0.6
Fewer children/higher quality	2	0	2	0.6
Pre-eclampsia	1	1	2	0.6
Other reasons (see below)	10	3	13	4.3
Total	139	35	174	
Negative				
Litigation (defensive medicine)	122	31	153	46.8
Misinterpretation of fetal monitoring results	12	6	18	5.5
Staffing problems (e.g. poor labour ward management)	14	1	15	4.6
Induction of labour	7	8	15	4.6
Unnecessary breech	2		2	0.6
Too active management of labour	2		2	0.6
Other (see below)	13	2	15	4.6
Total	172	48	220	
Total responses	565	155	720	
Total respondents			327	

are performing caesareans because they are frightened of being sued if anything goes wrong, rather than because it is the treatment that best suits the needs of mother and baby.

Table 8.1 shows that there were a total of 720 responses given by the 327 doctors replying to the question. This is an average of over two per consultant. They were more likely to mention positive rather than negative reasons for the increase in the caesarean rate by a ratio of three to two.

In analysing the results, we had to make some judgements regarding to which category to allocate a reason. For example, some consultants said that parents always wanted a perfect child, and others that they personally wanted to reduce risks to the baby. We have therefore separated them, although for some purposes they could be combined together with other reasons such as 'reduce the risk of brain damage'.

We found that there were contrasting attitudes towards electronic fetal monitoring which was mentioned overall by three in ten of the doctors. Some consultants were very positive towards it and made comments such as 'monitoring enables us to identify babies at risk'. Others, however, made comments such as that there was 'misinterpretation of fetal monitoring results' or, as a consultant from South East Thames stated, 'too much monitoring and too little facts'. A third group specified that fetal monitoring was a reason for the increase in caesareans without stating whether or not they approved of the change. A doctor from the Northern Region told of the 'routine use of fetal monitors in labour'. It is not clear whether the doctor was opposed to the practice. Because of this, such comments were placed in the category of 'neutral' reasons.

We initially put the ten comments about carrying out a caesarean in place of a forceps delivery into the neutral category. We know from our previous surveys that, as caesareans have increased, there has been a decline in the percentage of assisted deliveries by forceps.[5] However, in the end, we felt it fairer to place it with the other positive reasons, as many of them may be carried out because a caesarean is sometimes safer or may lead to less morbidity. In 1983 a consultant from the Northern Region wrote to us with a very instructive quote:

> It took three judicial hearings before damages of £100,000 were set aside (Jo Jordan case). The unpleasant publicity in the national press had all to be faced before the House of Lords ruled that an error of judgement did not amount to professional

---

5 Boyd and Francome, 1983; Francome, 1990b.

negligence. Should I produce a brain damaged baby by forceps delivery in 1983, that child can accuse me of negligence in a court of law until the year 2004. It is a worrying fact to face each time I am called to deal with the arrest of the head in the second stage of labour. I like to think it does not unduly influence my clinical judgement.[6]

Consultants in our recent survey made similar points. One from the North West Thames Region commented: 'There's been a change in indications and a caesarean is now a safer delivery rather than a difficult forceps.'

However, we should also recognise that the decline in using forceps may be partly because doctors are losing the skill as fewer forceps deliveries are carried out and the older practitioners with experience retire. The steady rise in popularity of Ventouse as a gentler alternative to forceps may also have contributed to the overall decline in their use. As a consultant from the Northern Region stated: 'Obstetricians are becoming more reluctant to undertake potentially difficult deliveries. With lack of experience this trend will accelerate. Although they find many statistical arguments to support this change, I am sure an underlying fear of litigation is a major factor.'

The positive reasons

The major positive reason was that improved care had increased the fetal survival rates, so in some cases doctors will now carry out a caesarean as a premature baby is more likely to survive. A crucial area of change is the care of premature babies, and consultants said that in some cases they would now carry out a caesarean when, previously, the baby would die in the womb undelivered or during the course of labour as it would be too immature to survive after birth, even if delivered by caesarean. As we shall discuss later, we did ask further questions on this issue.

A second important improvement is safety. This was identified as a factor by one in five of the obstetricians and almost half of these specified the increased safety of anaesthesia. Typical comments were: 'More likely to do for the baby now that the mother's risk is less.' A doctor from the Northern Region commented: 'There is increased safety of elective epidural section over the trial of labour for mother and baby.' Others mentioned such things as availability of epidural anaesthesia and the greater efficacy of antibiotics. A doctor in the East Midlands Region said there was 'increased safety of a caesarean, due to the development of obstetric anaesthesia and its use in

....

6 Boyd and Francome, 1983, p. 14.

preference to a vaginal delivery for primip breech, brow presentation and similar cases.'

The third most often mentioned positive reason was increased expectations of the parents. This was identified as important by 11.3 per cent of the obstetricians and the view of some was that the demand for a perfect baby is paramount. One doctor said that parents sometimes would not accept that his judgement of the balance of risks was right when the outcome was adverse.

In addition, 10.4 per cent mentioned the use of the operation to reduce morbidity of the baby and a further 5.5 per cent said to reduce perinatal mortality. Only 6.4 per cent made positive comments about electronic fetal monitoring. This is remarkably low, given its very widespread use.

Five consultants specified that they had a wish to reduce the risks of brain damage. A doctor from the West Midlands said that the increase was due to a 'Fear of a physical brain damage leading to earlier recourse to caesarean in fetal distress, prolonged labour and breech presentation.' This group was relatively small, however, and may be due to the fact that the earlier increase in caesareans in the period before 1970 did much to diminish this problem. Also, it is now known that only about 10 per cent of cases of cerebral palsy are due to events occurring in labour.

The neutral reasons

In this group, the largest category were those who simply mentioned electronic fetal monitoring without saying whether they were in favour of or opposed to its use. For example, a doctor from the North Western Region simply said 'Electronic monitoring' and many others followed suit. From this comment it is not clear whether the consultant approved or disapproved of the way fetal monitoring was being generally used. However, elsewhere we discuss this issue more fully (page 133).

The second highest reported factor in this group was breech delivery. Again most doctors did not specify whether they approved of the change or not and those few that did were largely divided. A consultant from South East Thames said: 'There has been a change in the pattern for breech presentation.' However, a doctor from Trent was much more positive: 'There is improved survival for premature breeches delivered by caesarean when less than 1,500 grams.' The fact that only one consultant in seven (14.7 per cent) mentioned breech is a large change from 1983 when it was mentioned by over two in five (41 per cent) and was the reason most often mentioned. The scientific validity for delivering breech babies by caesarean is a matter for debate. The only randomised controlled trial at term showed no difference in outcome for babies, but higher morbidity for women.[7] The higher morbidity for mothers was confirmed by Hofmeyr in an article supporting external cephalic version at term.[8] His article, however, suggests that the evidence supports improved outcome for the baby.

A total of sixteen consultants drew attention to the effects of the active management of labour. One said that 'It is better to have errors of commission than omission', and another said that 'there was a more active approach to long labour'. In addition to the reasons given by several doctors, there were thirteen different neutral reasons which were only mentioned by one consultant. These minor reasons are, however, of interest and include 'The realisation that caesarean is swift', 'We face pressure from paediatricians' and 'The fall in parity [number of births] has increased pressure.'

Thus we can see that there were many reasons given for the increase in caesarean rates which could not be clearly identified as due to improvements in practice.

The negative reasons

Almost half (46.8 per cent) of the consultants mentioned the use of caesarean to prevent litigation. This is a large increase over the percentage that identified this in our survey in 1983 when it was mentioned by less than a third of doctors (28.1 per cent). We found that the Jo Jordan case was mentioned by many in 1983 but in this study more recent cases seemed to be of concern. One doctor from the Northern Region stated: 'Litigation fears have grown since 1986'; while a Welsh doctor put the rise down to 'Ian Donald's book "Practical Obstetric Problems" ' (a book published in the 1950s). This intervention of the legal process into good medical practice is clearly a problem which has still to be resolved. When carrying out research for the 1990 study, Colin Francome received the following comments from a West Country obstetrician:

> Incidentally, I saw your name on a Maternity Alliance question form that one of my colleagues has completed. He says that the caesarean section rate has gone up because we are operating on smaller and smaller babies and that this has caused the salvage rate to go up. I am afraid the gentleman who filled up the form is utterly deluded. Our caesarean rate has gone up 300 percent in the fifteen years since I have been here and yet the salvage of small babies has not changed one jot. The reasons that the caesa-

7 Collea, Chein and Quilligan, 1980.
8 Hofmeyr, 1991.

rean section rate is going up is that we are all scared stiff of litigation.[9]

A doctor from the Wessex Region was similarly concerned about the change in attitude to litigation. He said that the reason for the increase in caesareans was entirely medico-legal, and stated somewhat poetically:

Instant perfection is the order of the day,
If not either then someone will pay.

He continued by commenting: 'The public will get what it deserves if it does not trust the medics to do their best.'

The second most frequently mentioned negative reason was that there was a misreading of fetal monitors and this was referred to by 5.5 per cent of the consultants. For example, one from Wales stated: 'There is uncertainty regarding the interpretation of monitoring in labour with a contribution due to fear of litigation.' Similarly a doctor from South East Thames said: 'There is too much monitoring, too little facts and no fetal blood sampling as routine.' This comment refers to the fact that if there are problems showing up on a monitor, they can be confirmed or otherwise by testing the fetal blood.

Fifteen consultants mentioned staffing problems. On this question there was not much unanimity, but instead a variety of different points were made. One mentioned less experienced labour ward staff; four said there were problems with junior doctors – they were either inexperienced or of deteriorating quality; one mentioned poorly trained middle-grade staff; and one said that registrars came mainly from overseas and showed less initiative in managing labour. A final comment was that the consultants' workload had tripled over the period. The number of consultants in England and Wales gives a ratio of one consultant to 800 births; in Scotland the ratio is about one to 500. Both figures are much lower than in the United States, where there are fewer midwives. The Royal College of Obstetricians and Gynaecologists' guidelines recommend a ratio of one doctor to 500 women, but some evidence shows that the higher the ratio of consultants to women, the higher the caesarean rate.[10]

There were other negative comments. Two said that the management of labour had become too active and the same number said there were too many caesareans for dystocia (long labour). Sixteen reasons were mentioned only once. These included 'Lack of knowledge about physiology of child-

9 Francome, 1990a, pp. 31–2.
10 Health Committee, 1992, pp. 74–5.

birth', 'Diminished expertise in operative deliveries' and 'caesareans are an easy option'.

Overall, the fact that more comments are positive than negative is heartening although, as we have seen, some of these reasons could be interpreted differently. It is also clear that from the point of view of many consultants, many caesareans were carried out unnecessarily.

British consultants' views of the caesarean rate in the United States

We have seen that the British consultants gave more positive than negative reasons for the rise in caesareans but it is also of interest to see how they viewed the much greater rise in the United States. We therefore asked the following question: 'The United States had a caesarean rate of 24.8% in 1987 and many hospitals had rates over 30%. What do you think are the major reasons for this?' Once we had excluded those who did not answer or said they did not know, this question was answered by 321 doctors. Of these, 278 stated litigation or legal factors as the reasons. Thus nearly nine British doctors out of ten (87 per cent) gave the fear of being sued as a reason. The second highest reason given was private practice, mentioned by forty-six consultants which is one in seven (14.3 per cent) of the sample. A doctor from the North Western Region gave this as a reason and then commented: 'There is a difference between private and public caesarean rates.' The evidence which we present on page 47 supports this view. The third highest reason given was 'patient pressure', and this seems to have been thought to be an important factor by thirty-three (10.3 per cent) of the British doctors. Almost as important as a reason was money, given by thirty-one (9.7 per cent) doctors. On this issue some pointed to the fact that where doctors are paid to attend all the births of women under their care, performing a caesarean helps them get to the next birth, or elsewhere, more quickly.

There were a variety of other explanations besides these which are of interest. Some mentioned the adage in the United States of 'once a caesarean, always a caesarean', and others the fact that in the United States midwives are rarely used to attend even normal deliveries. Finally a consultant from the Northern Region commented: 'The more caesareans you do the less able is the obstetrician to conduct a safe vaginal delivery.'

In Chapter 4 we mentioned the Task Force which the US government set up to consider the rise in the caesarean rates. This suggested that breech (15 per cent), repeat caesarean (27 per cent) and dystocia (29 per cent) had been responsible for tripling the rate between 1970 and 1978. Interestingly, the major reasons identified by the Task Force were rarely mentioned by the British obstetricians, so we could ask whether the British obstetricians were projecting what they understood to be the real reason for the rise in British rates onto the US rates.

Electronic fetal monitoring

Obstetricians believe fetal monitoring to be an important reason for the increased caesarean rate; however, it is not always clear why they considered it to be so. During the early days of their introduction in 1978, some doctors in New York complained to us that their colleagues began using them without adequate training in interpretation. One likened it to the early days of aircraft travel when there were initially many accidents. He felt that in a few years doctors would learn how to use the machines and there would be fewer unnecessary caesareans based on false interpretations. Others pointed out the need for fetal scalp blood sampling for confirmation of fetal distress.

The consultants in our survey were asked: 'Do you monitor all women electronically in labour?' The results (Table A8, page 182) show that just under half of all consultants in Britain monitored all women and that the practice was similar north and south of the Scottish border. Many consultants made further comments. Some followed the practice of the South West Thames respondent who said he 'monitored for 20 minutes at the start of labour'. Fifteen said that they monitored routinely for thirty minutes on arrival. A typical comment came from a Northern Region consultant: 'We routinely monitor all low risk patients for 30 minutes on admission and all high risk women until delivery.' Others did not state how long they would monitor all women. Hence a Wessex consultant said: 'We monitor all women on admission and then as necessary.' Others said that they monitored all women but only intermittently. For example, two said they monitored 'twenty minutes every two hours if everything was OK'. A consultant

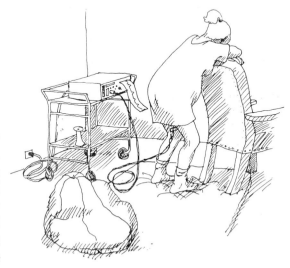

from North West Thames said: 'We *try* to monitor all (policy) but does anyone achieve 100% success?'

Those saying that they did not monitor routinely were further asked: 'What are your criteria for monitoring?' The results (Table A9, page 182) show that the major reason for monitoring was for 'high-risk' babies and this accounted for half of the responses. Furthermore, many of the other reasons given are a further specification of this. However, the definition of high risk is variable between doctors, with some classifying most of their population as high risk and others only a few.

Thirteen of the consultants said they took the mother's or parents' views into account. This was in some cases where they wanted to be monitored and in other cases where they objected to it. Some said they monitored all if a machine was available. A few consultants mentioned the role of the midwives in deciding whether there were sufficient problems for the use of the monitor. It was also evident that the woman was more likely to be monitored if she had been induced because of the risk of fetal distress caused by artificially strengthened contractions.

Under the 'other' reasons, a number of different comments were made. One mentioned prolonged labour and another 'women who are not in normal labour at term'. Other reasons given were that the woman was having her first baby, that she had a poor obstetric history and that she had pregnancy complications.

These responses are not easy to interpret, but suggest that there is no consensus of opinion among obstetricians. Women may be able to negotiate if they have enough information and are able to be assertive.

No-fault compensation

The most important negative reason suggested by consultants for the increase in the caesarean rates both in their own practice and overall in Britain was the fear of litigation. This may mean that many caesareans are being performed unnecessarily because doctors are scared of being sued.

A possible solution to this problem is no-fault compensation. Consultants were asked: 'Do you think that no-fault compensation for the parents of brain-damaged infants should be introduced?' The results (Table A10, page 183) showed that over four out of five (83.6 per cent) of consultants agreed with the introduction of no-fault compensation for the parents of brain-damaged babies. A doctor from the Yorkshire Region said: 'It should be made available via the National Health Service and the Department of Social Security.' A doctor from Wales supported the giving of compensation but said that it should not be a lump sum.

These issues are complex. Are the needs of a disabled child who suffers brain damage because of obstetric mismanagement different from one that resulted from a more naturally occurring disorder? One point we would like to make is that all parents with disabled babies need a great deal of help, and state provision varies widely from one locality to another. Where few facilities such as residential care or respite care are available, families have to take on many more responsibilities than in areas with better provision.

CARE FOR THE WOMAN DURING LABOUR
Time limit to labour

In post-war years there have been a number of consultants who do not feel that women should endure long labours. The policies of active management of labour initiated in Ireland (see pages 56–57) are well known and in Britain the definition of what is a long labour has come down from the eighteen-hour time demarcation of the British Birth Survey of 1970.[11] We asked consultants the following question: 'Do you have a time limit in labour after which a caesarean is normally performed?' The results (Table A11, page 183) showed that 88.6 per cent of the consultants had no time limit after which they would normally perform a caesarean. A doctor from the South Western Region said: 'It is based upon progress and is not about time.' A second from East Anglia said the decision 'depends on uterine activity', and a third from the Northern Region said: 'We have no rigid policy, it depends entirely on fetal-maternal condition.' A second consultant from the Northern Region said: 'The decision depends on progress including the strength of the contractions.' A consultant from the North Western Region said: 'Each individual is assessed if there is a failure to progress after four hours.'

Of those who did specify a time limit, a consultant from South West Thames said he would carry out a caesarean 'between 14–18 hours if there was no progress'. A Welsh doctor said he would conduct a 'critical review after 12 hours', while one from East Anglia specified '12 hours and no progress'. Thus there were a few doctors who said that they took account of the time, but they were a small minority compared to those who claimed to look at the whole of the labour in question.

Being awake for the caesarean

The consultants were asked: 'What proportion of caesareans are done under epidural in your firm?' Evidence from the previous chapter has shown that women are often pleased to be awake during their caesarean

....

11 Chamberlain and Chamberlain, 1975.

operation. This has the advantages that the woman is able to see the baby as soon as it is born, she is likely to feel much more involved in the proceedings and can usually have her labour companion with her. Women having general anaesthesia often report sadness at missing the birth.

The results showed (Table A12, page 183) that few consultants had accurate data about epidural rates and most of them estimated the percentage of operations done by this method. One in ten consultants rarely used an epidural for a caesarean, with 10 per cent of caesarean deliveries or fewer being done with the woman awake. However, at the other end of the scale, more than two in five consultants (43.5 per cent) said that an epidural was used in the majority of operations and some reported that nine out of ten operations were carried out in this way. One factor which influenced the use of epidural was whether the caesarean was elective or not. For example, a doctor from South West Thames said he used an epidural in 80 per cent of elective caesareans but only 30 per cent of emergency ones.

One factor which may affect the number of caesareans for which women are awake is the availability of epidural anaesthesia. Some hospitals only perform elective caesareans on certain days of the week when a suitably skilled anaesthetist is available to give epidurals. At other times, general anaesthesia is available for emergency caesareans, but epidurals are not available even when there is time to perform them before an emergency caesarean or for routine pain relief.

Partner's attendance at a caesarean

Most emergency caesareans are done by experienced staff in consultants' teams, not by the consultants personally, so their policies are important. The consultants were asked: 'Is the woman's partner invited to theatre for caesarean births?' We had answers to this from 347 consultants. Just under half (47.8 per cent) said they were invited, a slightly higher percentage (48.4 per cent) said they were sometimes invited and 3.7 per cent said they were not invited. Those who said that they sometimes invited the woman's partner to be present for the operation were asked what the decision depended upon, and we received a variety of replies.

A respondent from the Northern Region said he would invite the partner 'unless there were contra-indications such as a general anaesthetic'. Similarly a consultant from Wales said: 'I always invite the husband if we are using an epidural but would not usually for general anaesthetic.' In fact, for those who did place restrictions, the use of a spinal or epidural anaesthetic was by far the most common precondition. Among the other reasons, one Northern Region doctor said he would allow the observer 'If it was the woman's wish and it was not an emergency caesarean for fetal distress.' A second from the West Midlands Region had two preconditions for the partner's attendance: that 'the caesarean was elective and under epidural'. Another doctor from the Trent Region said: 'It is up to the surgeon, the anaesthetist and midwifery staff at the time to decide.'

One of the few doctors to say he would not invite the partner into the theatre nevertheless commented: 'I do not invite the partner to observe but if the patient requests attendance then I usually agree.' So apart from this comment, there seem to be a very small number of doctors who will not allow the partner to attend under any conditions, at least in theory. However, in practice, if the labour ward is busy, the partner may not be invited unless he and the woman ask.

CONCLUSION

When considering the responses of the consultants to our questionnaire, the most striking comments are those on the reasons for the increase in caesarean rates. The fact that they sometimes mentioned such factors as litigation, misinterpretation of electronic fetal monitoring results and staffing problems shows that there is an urgent need for improvements in care. In Chapter 5 we discussed the indications for caesarean based on problems that might occur for the woman or the 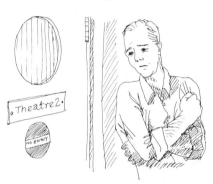 baby. It is changes in research-based knowledge of these kinds of indication that should determine alterations in the caesarean rate, not concerns about legal action or a shortage of staff.

The increase in concern about litigation in recent years is a particularly worrying trend. It means that doctors are not free to make their judgements and present the evidence to women in the most objective light but have to be concerned about possible legal effects. Even more worrying is the influence on consultant practice of ill-informed lawyers who insist on evidence provided by traces from electronic fetal monitors in respect of all women, not just those who are regarded as being at higher risk.[12]

....

12 Giesen, 1993.

To have a brain-damaged baby for whatever reason is bound to cause real hardship for families. We suggest that the consultants' pleasingly overwhelming desire for no-fault compensation should lead to serious consideration of new ways of helping families provide for disabled children, whether or not there has been medical negligence.

There are difficulties with the use of electronic fetal monitoring. When monitors were first introduced, the traces were often misinterpreted and used without checking the results with the use of fetal blood sampling. This led to unnecessary caesarean operations. From the diversity of attitudes towards electronic fetal monitors among consultants, it is clear that there is confusion about how they should be used, if at all, in order to help improve diagnosis. This is in spite of good randomised controlled trials showing that electronic fetal monitoring results should always be checked using fetal blood sampling.[13]

With breech deliveries also there are questions as to how far a caesarean is necessary. It seems that the trend towards performing caesarean for breech began with little, if any, research to support it. This raises the issue of the way in which some practices come into being without any clear indications that they are an improvement.

On the positive side, the results of this survey taken over a two-year period with a good response rate provide some hope for improving care. It was only a few years ago that men were discouraged from attending even a normal delivery. Now they are usually able to be present at a caesarean performed under regional anaesthesia. This means that fathers are more likely to feel involved with their children and so take a more active role. Many consultants say that they take the parents' views into account on the question of an early caesarean for fetal distress and whether to monitor. Thus it seems that some attempt is being made to be responsive to parents' feelings and wishes, although we would recognise that many groups would feel that there is a long way to go in this direction.

....

13 MacDonald et al., 1985.

CHAPTER NINE

VAGINAL BIRTH AFTER CAESAREAN

Nothing could stop me now. I just could not have an elective caesarean knowing that there was no real reason. The consultant had other ideas, though. Even in view of this great news he still refused to agree a trial of labour.

WE have seen in our survey that only one in 100 consultants in England and Wales and four in 100 in Scotland support the policy of 'once a caesarean, always a caesarean'. However, our study also showed that few consultants are enthusiastic about a vaginal birth after caesarean (VBAC – pronounced 'veeback'). In a special issue on the subject, the Association for Improvements in the Maternity Services claimed that in Britain only about half of all women have a vaginal birth after caesarean despite the fact that only a minority of women have recurring reasons for one.[1] This suggestion is supported by our survey in which the majority of consultants allowed about half to three-fifths of the women to have vaginal deliveries. It would be possible to have a much higher average. In fact 5.6 per cent of consultants claimed that more than 80 per cent of women treated by their team had a VBAC. The level that might be achieved is illustrated by a series of 1,781 women who had a VBAC rate of 91 per cent. However, in part the VBAC rate was this high because 1,009 of the women had also had a previous vaginal delivery.[2]

In giving the view from the British obstetricians' perspective, Philipp states that all wounds leave scar tissue which has a different structure from the original, and sometimes it is stronger and on other occasions weaker.[3]

THE EVIDENCE ON SAFETY

An important piece of research reviewed the literature from 1950 to 1980 and found that out of 5,325 VBACs there was not a single maternal death related to uterine rupture. Although there were fourteen fetal

1 AIMS, 1991.
2 Molloy, Sheil and Duignan, 1987.
3 Philipp, 1988, p. 63.

deaths, twelve of these were due to the rupture of a prior classical scar. Only two fetal deaths were related to the rupture of a low transverse incision but both of these occurred before 1965 and in unmonitored women.[4] This evidence supports the view that a lower-segment section produces a much more resilient post-operative uterus. As we have seen, this view was first put forward in the 1920s (Chapter 3).

In a study of 353 women with a previous caesarean at Queen Charlotte's (London) Maternity Hospital from 1980 to 1987, a total of 158 were delivered by elective caesarean section. This left 195 who were allowed a trial of scar: of these, 79 per cent delivered vaginally while the others had emergency operations. There were two stillbirths in the series. One of these resulted from scar dehiscence in a mother whose labour was induced with two prostaglandin pessaries. The other stillbirth was due to the fetus having hydrocephaly and spina bifida. There were no neonatal deaths.[5] The production of extra-strong contractions during induced labour is a recognised potential problem.[6] In 1988 the Committee of Obstetrics of the American College of Obstetricians and Gynecologists drew attention to the potential risk of uterine rupture from the administration of oxytocin and pointed out that some physicians choose not to use it to induce or speed up labour in women who have undergone a prior caesarean. An Irish study of 2,176 consecutive cases of delivery after caesarean section found that oxytocin was only likely to increase the probability of scar rupture if used in conjunction with epidural anaesthesia. In this series a repeat elective section was performed on 395 mothers (18.2 per cent) and, of the rest, 90.8 per cent achieved a vaginal birth with only eight of the 1,781 women going into labour experiencing the rupture of the scar.[7] No babies died as a result of this.

Other international evidence comes from the Princess Margaret Hospital in Kowloon, Hong Kong. Over an eight-year period from 1976 to 1983 nearly 1,300 mothers were allowed to try for a VBAC. Not all women were allowed a trial of labour and the researchers specified four preconditions before a woman could attempt a VBAC:

1. Just one previous caesarean by lower-segment operation.
2. Information to be obtained about the previous caesarean including the reasons for it and progress after the operation.
3. There should be no likelihood of disproportion.

4 Lavin, Stephens, Miodovnik and Barden, 1982, p. 135.
5 Coltart, Davies and Katesmark, 1990, pp. 1140–3.
6 Placek, Taffel and Moien, 1988.
7 Molloy et al., 1987, p. 1645.

4. The woman should have a careful examination to make sure the head could engage. This would exclude breech deliveries, for example.

Three-quarters of the mothers had a successful VBAC whereas in many hospitals in the United States they would not even have been given the opportunity of a trial of labour. The authors of the study recognised that there is a risk of the scar rupturing in labour and indeed over the study period eleven women, not all of them in the study, did have scars that ruptured.[8] However, the authors maintain that even if a scar in the lower segment of the uterus does rupture, there is no great danger to the mother or baby. They confirm that only in women where the scar is the old-fashioned vertical one is the risk of rupture significant. This was for two reasons: first of all, a vertical scar was more likely to rupture because muscular activity is greater in the upper segment; and second, because the tear could extend both up and down and if it did so to a marked degree, the baby could move outside the uterus.

The lack of danger from rupture of the uterus was supported by the Canadian Consensus Conference on Aspects of Caesarean Childbirth. It was reported that in four series of VBAC studies over 2,000 births, the likelihood of scar rupture leading to an emergency delivery was only 0.2 per cent, whereas the frequency of other emergencies requiring an immediate caesarean in 11,800 non-VBAC births was 2.7 per cent.[9] Similarly, analysis of 1,156 emergency repeat caesareans during attempted VBAC in San Antonio found the frequency of scar rupture to be the very low figure of 0.09 per cent.[10]

In reviewing the evidence, Flamm argued recently that 'dozens of studies filled the medical literature with data supporting VBAC. But for many years their recommendations fell on deaf ears'.[11] Women, especially in the United States, continued to be told by doctors that if they attempted a VBAC they would be risking a brain-damaged baby or a hysterectomy. Other women were told that community hospitals were not equipped to deal with a VBAC.

In Ireland there is a much lower rate of first caesareans and so these women might be regarded as those with more potential problems than comparable mothers in the United States, where obstetricians are likely to perform a caesarean much more readily. Despite this, the VBAC rate in Ireland is estimated at 65–70 per cent.[12]

....

8 Lao, Leung and Young, 1987.
9 Canadian Conference, 1986.
10 Shearer, 1992.
11 Flamm, 1992, p. 31.
12 MacDonald, 1992, p. 32.

VAGINAL BIRTH AFTER TWO OR MORE CAESAREANS

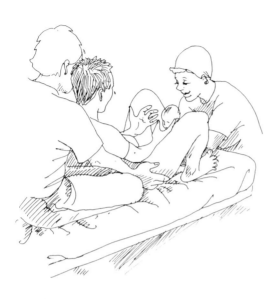

We have seen that the authors of the Hong Kong study regarded more than one previous caesarean as a contraindication for a vaginal delivery. However, an interesting piece of research on 1,000 women showed that 501 had a trial of labour after more than one caesarean, and of those women about 70 per cent delivered vaginally.[13] In a second study of 177 such women, while only 35 were allowed a trial of labour, nearly 4 out of 5 (77 per cent) of these had a vaginal delivery.[14] There was no increase in maternal or fetal mortality associated with labour, and although the study was small, the evidence also supports a trial of labour in mothers who have had more than one caesarean. Indeed there does not seem to be any reason that the scar should be any weaker after two caesareans than after one.

WOMEN'S EXPERIENCES OF VBAC
Case study 1: A pelvis just big enough

When Susan was thirty-nine weeks pregnant it was confirmed that her first baby was breech. Her obstetrician recommended pelvimetry and according to the X-ray, her pelvis was 'borderline' (9–10 cm and not roomy enough for a vaginal breech delivery). She was due to have an elective caesarean but before it was due, she entered spontaneous labour. She commented on her emergency caesarean that she was happy to have laboured as it gave her confidence for future deliveries. She had a son, Guy, and says that, while she was disappointed *'that my squatting practice, perineal massage and all the longed-for natural birth stuff had all been in vain . . . I could not doubt that the caesarean was the best course of action in this case'*. When she fell pregnant again she commented:

....

13 Phelan, Ahn and Diaz, 1989.
14 Hansell, McMurray and Huey, 1990, p. 146.

All through my second pregnancy I had doubts as to whether I was capable of a vaginal delivery and the thought of just going ahead and booking an elective caesarean did cross my mind a few times. However, I convinced myself to wait and see how the baby was presenting at term and go from there. My obstetrician (the same one as last time) is very caring and supportive and told me to go ahead and do what I felt was right and he would tell me if I was being foolhardy. What would be ideal was a head-down presentation and for everything to be spontaneous with the onset of labour, rupture of the membranes and delivery. I attended NCT classes again and practised squatting like mad; in front of the TV, washing machine and brushing the dog, so really my pelvis would have no excuse. As term approached, my baby was head-down which was much different from last time and I could breathe.

At thirty-eight weeks and five days, I started labour very slowly but surely one Sunday evening. I realised vaguely that I was having slight pains exactly ten minutes apart but as I was nine days from the due date I ignored them and went to bed. By midnight they were strong enough to wake me and at 5.00 a.m. I phoned the midwives at the hospital. Considering my history, they asked me to go in straight away and when I arrived the contractions were three minutes apart and getting stronger.

My obstetrician examined me at 8.00 a.m. and said I would probably be delivered by lunchtime, possibly with forceps. He also fitted me up with a cannula in my wrist in case of uterine rupture and the need to get blood into me fast. My membranes ruptured spontaneously and by 9.00 a.m. I couldn't move off the bed and I was lying on my side with the TENS machine blasting away, so my squatting plan was up the shoot. Suddenly at 9.35 a.m. I started pushing. It was spontaneous and felt a little bit like retching but at the other end. Cecily was born at 9.40 a.m. with no drugs, no stitches and no problems. Aren't I lucky?

Case study 2: A VBAC at home   Gina Lowden of Hampshire gave us permission to tell of her experiences. Her first baby arrived after a long labour ending in an emergency caesarean with an epidural. The baby was breech and she felt that a caesarean was inevitable. She comments on her second delivery:

Having always wanted to have my babies at home for some deep and unknown reason, among the many tears I shed following the section were some because I thought I wouldn't be able to have my second baby at home. Then I started to wonder why not? Some two years later I came to the conclusion that there were no valid medical or physical reasons why I couldn't give birth at home perfectly safely. In fact when I weighed up the pros and cons, it was very clear to me that in my case at least, it was in all probability safer for me to have my second baby at home.

She went on to say that she expected opposition from the medical staff and was not convinced of the value of early antenatal care. She did not contact her local hospital to explain her reasons for wanting a home delivery until she was twenty weeks and the hospital set up a meeting with a community midwife at her home. She was ready to have an 'out-and-out battle' but:

None came. She was wonderful. No arguments. No lectures on the risks, no attempt at emotional blackmail. She explained that I would not be able to be offered continuity of care because of staffing levels, which was a big disappointment, but she assured me that none of her midwives would try and 'get me in', and I believed she spoke the truth and was not wool-pulling. She also wanted me to ensure that I was happy to have my antenatal care from the local community midwives.

Her home delivery was fixed and so she decided to tell her local GP out of courtesy and to ask for his agreement to provide emergency cover. She said that she expected him either to treat her as a silly girl or to be threatening, but '*the poor man simply fell apart in front of me*'. She felt that the sheer responsibility of what he felt to be a near-fatal course of events was almost too much for him. However, he wrote to her agreeing to give the cover and suggested that she went to the local hospital to see the consultant. She decided against that course of action as she had been told that the consultant was opposed to VBAC and she wanted to avoid unnecessary conflict. Gina records the birth as follows:

On 18 February, some ten days before my due date, I woke up with a sharp pain in my pubic bone area. It only lasted a moment and was accompanied by a little trickle of water. I went downstairs to the loo and the contractions came thick and fast. Gordon, my husband, came to see what was going on, realised I was in labour and said 'What do we do now?' 'Oh, nothing yet' I said, thinking it would be hours. He went away but I was wrong. Shortly afterwards I had two contractions that I found very difficult to cope with. The 'water buffalo' noises I was making brought Gordon back quickly. I remembered reading in Grantly Dick-Read's book Childbirth without Fear *that you never have more than ten like that before you're in the second stage and pushing. I was incredulous, surely it couldn't be that fast.*

Suddenly I wanted the reassurance of a midwife and started shouting instructions at Gordon: phone the hospital, the number is by the phone, the labour ward number, tell them it's definitely labour, tell them it's going fast, tell them I think I can feel the head. Then poor Gordon had to run around preparing upstairs. There were things that needed to be moved. Then a stream of further instructions as to where to put the dustbin bags down as I had not acquired a polythene sheet, and where to find the old sheet to put on top. It was different for Gordon this time too – no time to get bored, no long hours spent trying to doze in an uncomfortable hospital chair.

As soon as he'd finished I removed upstairs. Immediately the next contraction ended in a definite push. There was nothing I could do, my body was pushing and that was that. Where's the midwife! The poor girl arrived in a panic. The first on-call midwife lived an hour's drive away, and as she was much nearer, she got the call and been told we could see the head. Then she'd been unable to find the house. Gordon had spotted her running to the phone box outside and had gone to get her. She discovered I was fully dilated and satisfied herself the baby was head-down and not breech. I suggested that one of the community midwives who'd given me antenatal care might be prepared to come as back-up and she ran downstairs to phone. It was now 7.00 a.m. just two hours after I had woken up.

From then on it all went like clockwork. The local midwife arrived in minutes, the atmosphere in the room calmed down. With each other for support, the two midwives were wonderful, although I was so busy I really did not pay them much heed. Pushing was painful. It brought tears to my eyes. I was offered gas and air and knew there was pethidine in the fridge, but I did not want pain relief. It's not that I'm a martyr or anything, but I was too busy concentrating to be bothered with the distraction. I was on my knees with my perineum on the floor leaning forward over a very low stool – not the most wonderful position for giving birth. The midwives were unsuccessfully trying to coax me into a more advantageous position. The urges to push got stronger and then I got a bit between my teeth and decided I had had enough and this baby was coming out.

I pushed through the pain. Too late the midwife called 'pant'. His head was out. Moments later during the same contraction his body slithered out. It was 7.45 a.m., less than three hours since I'd woken up. I collapsed with exhaustion. I had absolutely no energy left. There were cries of 'Mummy, it's a baby, Mummy, it's a boy.' My daughter, who was a month away from her fourth birthday, chose to be present. I'm not sure how she reacted really. I don't think she was frightened. She was with her dad who was happy to sit back and let the midwives do their stuff. I'm glad she chose to be there, as she has seen birth as a normal life event, and didn't have to be separated from her mum which she would have found difficult to cope with.

My GP visited the first day to carry out the paediatric check and put me in mind of a dog with two tails. 'You proved them all wrong, didn't you!' he greeted me. 'I told you I would,' I replied. Of that I have never been in any doubt, even though I could see close friends thinking I might be over-confident. When it comes to having babies, a woman can't be over-confident.

Case study 3: Two caesareans followed by two vaginal births

Sheridan Brown told of her experiences more fully in a special issue on VBAC in the *AIMS Journal*.[15] She explained that her first birth, of Peter, was by emergency caesarean after thirty-four hours of labour. She was the 'perfect patient' who did exactly as she was told and did not question any decisions made on her behalf. In 1988 she was pregnant again and her routine scan at sixteen weeks showed full placenta praevia which had not changed by thirty-eight

---

15 AIMS, 1991.

weeks, so she had an elective caesarean. She found it difficult to bond with her daughter, Honor, at first but after about three days *'a wave of love just swept over me'*. In January 1990, when pregnant a third time, at thirteen weeks she asked a hospital doctor if a vaginal delivery would be possible and whether she could have four babies by caesarean. She and her husband had always wanted four children and she was given a negative response to both questions; she relates further events as follows:

> *I was devastated. I went home and wrote a very depressed letter to the Caesarean Support Network and then set about trying to come to terms with, and prepared myself for what I could see, as an inevitable section. In May I got a telephone call from Yvonne Williams. We spent a long time discussing the risk of uterine rupture and my right to have a vaginal delivery if I so wished. It sounds odd, but I just hadn't thought that I could have any say in what happened to me. What Yvonne told me and the information she subsequently posted to me sent me scurrying to the library where I waded through countless British Medical Journals and made a note of any relevant studies. My battle had begun. At this point I must stress that I am just an ordinary wimp. I don't like even taking goods back to a shop for fear of making a scene.*
>
> *Over the next few weeks I worked very hard. I had numerous confrontations with my consultant and his entourage. Each time came the firm instruction they were absolutely against me having even a trial of labour. I could not believe that in view of all the information I had come across regarding the risk of uterine rupture (actually around 0.7%) and the associated risk of a repeat caesarean (around 2–11%), that the obstetrician considered it better (or more convenient?) to take the greater risk of repeat caesarean section rather than at least try for a vaginal delivery.*
>
> *One of the biggest issues with my consultant was the fact that, according to pelvimetry I had when pregnant with Honor, I had a smallish pelvis. I agreed to have a scan at 37 weeks. My smallest measurement was my pelvic outlet which was 10.5cm. The scan showed the baby's head was 8.9cm. I was overjoyed. Nothing could stop me now. I just could not have an elective caesarean knowing that there was no real reason. The consultant had other ideas, though. Even in view*

of this great news he still refused to agree a trial of labour. By now we had made our decision and nothing in the world could change our resolve.

At 3am on Sunday 26th August 1990 (38 weeks), I awoke with mild stomach ache. By 3.30am I realised I must be in labour, but decided to go back to bed as I had two false alarms the previous week. I soon discovered that the pain was far greater lying down and so I got up and had some breakfast. I got the children's things organised and packed my labour bag. My contractions were already coming at about seven minute intervals – although very short, about thirty seconds. Even though they were quite intense, because they were short, they were relatively easy to deal with.

Allan awoke at 5am and prepared me a bath. That was lovely. We decided to time the contractions and they were coming every 4–5 minutes, but still very short. Allan suggested we ring my parents so they could come to look after the children. My parents arrived at 7.00am but I was afraid of going into hospital too early, was still unsure whether the time was right. My contractions were coming every 3–4 minutes but I was able to deal with them and therefore presumed I was not in established labour. Allan eventually persuaded me to go in and so we set off on the 5 minute journey and I was admitted about 7.30am. I agreed to have an external monitor and remained standing as this was the most comfortable position. The midwife who admitted me said I was about 2–3cm dilated – this confirmed my fear that we had gone in too early.

At about 7.45am the nursing shifts changed and in walked a midwife I knew. She was very supportive and I felt I could completely trust her – that helped a great deal. The registrar came in at 8.00am and said she must advise me to have a section – after a short, very good humoured discussion, where I assured her I understood the risks, which were minimal as I saw it, and I still wanted to try, she accepted that. I knew she was just trying to cover herself and establish that I knew what I was doing. She was not at all pushy. She gave me an internal examination. Then she gave me Entonox to help with the pain. When I heard I was 6cm dilated I was ecstatic.

During the first examination my membranes ruptured and the pain increased considerably so I decided to have an epi-

dural. The anaesthetist arrived at about 9.00am and did a very quick and painless job of it. He had just given me a very small test amount and was just taping the catheter up my back when I gave a little grunt and pushed. The midwife asked the anaesthetist to delay the main dose and examined me – I was 10cm dilated only an hour after my first examination. In fact just that first dose of epidural was perfect. I had complete abdominal pain relief, but had full sensation vaginally. I knew exactly when I wanted to push and could feel the baby moving down the birth canal.

Even though I was dilated to 10cm, there was still a small lip and I could not push for a few minutes. At that point a woman came into the room. I knew she was the consultant on duty. After a few minutes of watching silently she said abruptly 'I hope you realise that even at this stage you could still have a brain damaged baby'. Allan looked at her and said 'but it would still be loved'. There was a pause and then she said 'I hope you don't ruin the next four hours of my day.' With that she left the room. Fortunately I was expecting more opposition and was well prepared mentally so at the time her comments went over my head. But now in retrospect, I see that these few words, and their timing, could have completely destroyed someone and were inexcusable. I am complaining.

I was ready to begin the second stage and found the traditional semi-upright sitting position to be very comfortable. Allan had been very supportive until this stage but now he really shone. He was right down at my 'business end' with my left foot on his hip, holding my hand and wiping my face with a damp cloth. He was absolutely brilliant and as the midwife told me what to do, Allan reiterated it and I responded to his voice, it was real teamwork. After ten minutes of pushing the registrar came back and suggested she 'just lift the baby out with a pair of forceps'. I politely refused. The midwife stepped in and said 'Let's let this lady go for a normal delivery shall we?' The registrar stepped back and let the midwife do her job.

Eventually I got more of a hang of pushing and things got really moving. Allan told me to reach down and feel the baby's head. The first time it still felt a long time inside, but the second time it felt like it was almost out and it gave me impetus to carry on. The baby's head was born and I was surprised at how big his shoulders felt inside. With the next push he was delivered on to my stomach. It was a boy. I was on a mountain top – 'I did it', 'I did it', I exclaimed over again. I loved him immediately. It was one of the most satisfying and great moments of my life. We called him Jakke. I showed him my breast and he licked it a bit, but he wasn't really interested – it didn't matter – I had my baby in my arms, all bloody and slippy and wide awake.

After this birth she had another vaginal delivery.

Case studies 4 and 5: Painful VBACs   The women in the first three examples were very keen to have a vaginal birth after caesarean and we can admire their courage and fortitude in the face of great difficulties. Other women may have a VBAC without the same enthusiasm and in the interests of balance it is instructive to consider the views of two other women.

Norma, a schoolteacher in the horseracing town of Lambourn, said that she did not really enjoy either of her births but overall preferred the vaginal delivery. In her first birth she had not dilated after thirty-two hours in labour. She went into labour at 8.00 p.m. on a Wednesday about two weeks before her due date. The waters broke and she was given a drip. *'I didn't know what was in it, I just let them get on with it. They decided on the caesarean about five o'clock on the Friday morning. Then they waited so as not to disturb the doctor too early. So I had David at 7.30 a.m. and for the first day I was too drowsy to bother with him.'*

She did not ask for a vaginal birth for her second delivery and when it came she was not prepared for the pain:

> *I only had gas and air as I did not ask for any pain relief early enough. I was screaming so loud that the midwife threatened to take away even the gas and air. I can't help laughing about it now, but at the time I would have died if I could. However, once Matthew had been born I was fine. I took to him straight away and I was up around the ward giving out tea the next day.*

Viv Williamson has three sons with the first being born by caesarean. *'I was in labour for forty-eight hours. I dilated only 3 cm. He was lying facing the wrong way and so he did not come down far enough to stimulate me to dilate.'* She had a caesarean without much problem and breastfed her son Jack for seven months.

> *After the caesarean I had to wander round stooped over like an old lady for a couple or three days. You're so terrified that the stitches are going to pull out if you stand up. I did my exercises with dedication. They were very gentle – lying on the bed and wiggling my toes and gentle sit-ups and was running in six weeks. I thought I would be a broken reed but I ran like an athlete. I wanted to have a vaginal birth the second time and I was in labour for seventeen hours. I found the first vaginal birth very painful and they cut me and I had to have stitches. I have quite narrow hips – about 32 inches. Because of the stitches the recovery was slower than it might have been. For my second vaginal birth the labour was only eight hours and it was no sweat – I was up and about.*

INFORMATION AND SUPPORT NETWORK FOR VBAC

We have seen from the academic data in this chapter and in Chapter 4 that there is a great deal of concern about VBAC within the medical profession. The case histories above show that the medical attitudes to individual pregnancies have left many women feeling that they have to do battle with the profession rather than work with it. The above examples show that some obstetricians have been seen to make cutting and unhelpful comments. This is unfortunate. Childbirth is a very significant event in parents' lives and it is of the utmost importance that the quality of care, both physical and emotional, is of the highest order. Women will then have good memories of their delivery and when each birthday of their child arrives, they can think back warmly to the important occasion and the support and help they received from those attending the birth.

The British groups supporting VBACs have produced an action plan for women. It reads as follows:

> Vaginal Birth after Caesarean Section is not easy or straightforward for anyone. If you feel strongly about it and would like to be successful, you are well advised to make a careful and thorough assessment of your own situation.
>
> A) Make sure you know the reason for your previous section(s).

B) Find out what your hospital's policies are, do they vary by consultant?

C) Find out what facts will adversely affect your chances of achieving a VBAC

- Continuous electronic fetal monitoring
- Restriction of food and fluid intake
- Restriction of mobility
- Acceleration of labour by ARM [artificial rupture of the membranes]
- Time limits
- Staff changes
- Induction or augmentation (acceleration of labour with oxytocin).

D) If you have, or have had, any one of the following you may find your hospital will be recommending a caesarean as routine:

- Cephalopelvic [feto-pelvic] disproportion
- Two or more previous caesarean sections
- Twins or breech
- Postdates
- A classical or T incision

E) Contact the lay organisations for information about achieving a VBAC next time. [See Further Information for Parents, page 198.]

We would like to add the following points:

- Take your time over choosing your hospital and/or your consultant: do not be rushed into a hasty decision.
- If you decide to change hospital from the previous time, ensure that your notes are obtained, together with the results of any X-rays taken after the caesarean.
- Prepare yourself mentally and physically for a VBAC and read Chapter 10 of this book, much of which is relevant to VBAC.

CHAPTER TEN

AVOIDING UNNECESSARY CAESAREANS

More information on choice of places for birth should be provided by the GP earlier. I had booked into one hospital on the advice of the GP as it was our 'local' hospital. At 24 weeks, I requested a change so I could use a more progressive hospital. The GP respected my wishes and I was transferred. The choice of hospitals should be made after Mum's given time to consider the options – rather than at the same time as receiving a positive pregnancy test.

Previous chapters have shown that caesareans are sometimes performed unnecessarily:

● There is wide variation in the caesarean rates between different maternity units which cannot be accounted for by different populations.
● Some of the indications for caesareans are relative rather than absolute. Even different obstetricians within the same maternity unit treat relative indications differently when deciding whether to advise a woman to have a caesarean.
● Although electronic fetal monitoring has become routine in many units, the accuracy of its interpretation remains extremely difficult and the results are not checked by fetal blood sampling as often as they should be.
● The relative safety of the modern caesarean, particularly when performed under regional anaesthesia, has become confused with medico-legal considerations to increase the readiness of obstetricians to perform caesareans sooner rather than later.

In our opinion, the current caesarean rate in Britain, shown by our sample to be 13 per cent, is too high. The aim of this chapter, therefore, is to show how some caesareans could be avoided. However safe and unthreatening the operation might become for women, nevertheless the post-operative recovery is never likely to be a positive addition to the first few weeks of looking after a new baby. Because maternity care works best when it is a team effort between each woman and her caregivers, we recommend all women and their caregivers to read this chapter in its entirety. Appendix A contains a table describing the principal features of different packages of maternity care.

CONTINUITY OF CARER

The more comfortable a woman feels with the place of birth and the people caring for her, the more likely it is that her birth will be straightforward. Being looked after by people with whom she has a good relationship will empower her to make informed choices. Increasingly, the emphasis in enlightened systems of maternity care aiming at the minimum number of medical interventions (and therefore only necessary caesareans) is on 'continuity of carer'. Continuity of carer can be defined for these purposes as each woman getting to know a small group of midwives responsible for her care during pregnancy, birth and postnatally. In particular, the midwife looking after the woman during labour will have got to know the woman during pregnancy and will be able to care for her according to her preferences. Even when women need medical assistance, they continue to receive much of their care from midwives. If the need for medical intervention is unexpected, the care of midwives known to the woman is of even more value than when labour progresses normally. Some GPs offer the whole package of maternity care, including care during labour, to their patients, but usually rely on community midwives to give much of the care. However, women usually receive a high level of continuity from this kind of arrangement, quite different from the usual 'shared care' package.

Much modern maternity care is fragmented, with many women being cared for by a large number of different health professionals during pregnancy, birth and afterwards:

> In itself, the overall number of health professionals may not be the most important factor of continuity of carer. A high number of carers does not rule out the opportunity for one midwife or doctor to be coordinating care and offering on-going support. However, the number of carers is a simple indicator of the likelihood of continuity of carer in view of the way services are currently organised for women.[1]

The NCT 1992 Maternity Services Survey found that 23 per cent of the respondents received care from twenty or more different health professionals; 40 per cent from ten to nineteen professionals; and 37 per cent from fewer than ten.[2]

....

1 Newburn, 1993.
2 Newburn, 1993.

Often nowadays the only way to achieve continuity of carer, particularly in urban areas, is for a woman to book a home birth or domino (see Appendix A). In rural areas, particularly those served by small maternity units, continuity of carer is more likely to happen because there are smaller numbers of both women and midwives so it is easier for them to get to know each other. In a few district health authorities, efforts are being made to improve continuity of carer as a result of the House of Commons Health Committee's report on maternity services published in 1992.

CHOOSING THE PACKAGE OF MATERNITY CARE

It is important for the woman not to be rushed into arranging her care for pregnancy and birth until she has had time to find out all the options available and to consider which package of care she feels is best. It is very common for a woman to visit her GP after a positive pregnancy test and be expected to decide on her care there and then. It was shown in letters sent in by women with their replies to the 1992 NCT Maternity Services Survey that GPs do not always inform women about all the available choices. This may be either because they are not aware of them or because there are certain options, such as total midwife care, for which they would not receive the usual item of service payment.

> More information on choice of places for birth should be provided by the GP earlier. I had booked into one hospital on the advice of the GP and it was our 'local' hospital. At 24 weeks, I requested a change so I could use a more progressive hospital. The GP requested my wishes and I was transferred. The choice of hospitals should be made after the Mum's given time to consider the options – rather than at the same time as receiving a positive pregnancy test.[3]

Other sources of information about options for care are the local branch of the NCT (see Further Information for Parents, page 198), community midwives (usually based at the nearest maternity unit), the community health council (in the telephone directory), family and friends. The table in Appendix A shows the basic features of each package of maternity care. In addition to options provided by the NHS, some women may wish and be able to afford to use an independent midwife or a private hospital.

....

3 National Childbirth Trust, 1992.

When looking into the local options, the woman can enquire about the approaches to care during pregnancy and birth and can also ask for up-to-date statistics as well as any other factors or facilities such as the availability of a birthing pool or special care baby unit. Caesarean rates can often be an indicator of a more or less technological approach to birth, but it is important to find out at the same time whether a unit with a substantially lower caesarean rate than another unit in the same health district is only caring for women at 'low risk' of complications during labour. Caesarean rates are often also linked to forceps and/or Ventouse rates so that if one is lower, the other may be higher. If a woman has a pre-existing medical condition or a difficult obstetric history, it is probably wise for her to discuss the implications for pregnancy and birth with an obstetrician and/or other medical specialist before deciding on her care.

If a woman intends to give birth in hospital, she can arrange to visit and be given a guided tour. This will provide an idea of the atmosphere of the maternity unit and the opportunity to ask questions informally. Since the recent NHS changes and the advent of the internal market, hospitals may be increasingly prepared to welcome women in this way, and some units organise regular weekly tours for this purpose.

In addition to the choices of place of birth, midwives and style of care, another variable a woman should take into account when choosing her care is the approach and policies of individual consultant obstetricians. As has been shown by our survey of consultants, their attitude to the management of labour can affect the chance of having a caesarean significantly. Informal sources of this information might include the senior midwife in charge of the hospital antenatal clinic and local branches of the NCT and AIMS. Other more direct sources would be the senior manager of maternity services or the clinical director. These data are collected and processed at the taxpayer's expense and should therefore be available to the public. Care should be taken in interpreting data as some consultants may specialise in high-risk cases. GPs may be able to help.

Once a woman has found out about all the local options for care and any special implications arising for her, she can consider which package feels right for her. If she has a partner, she may want to take his views into account, especially if he is going to be with her in labour. Alternatively, if the couple's attitudes to the place of birth differ, the woman may ask a friend or relative to be her labour companion.

CHOOSING A HOME BIRTH

In many ways, having a baby at home is the surest way of achieving continuity of carer, avoiding routine procedures and intervention, encouraging the normal progress of labour and thus minimising the risk of a caesarean. However, since childbirth in Britain has become medicalised, many women do not have confidence in their ability to give birth without medical supervision and therefore feel more secure labouring in hospital. We acknowledge this need and therefore welcome the trend to make hospitals more homely and welcoming to women and their labour companions and families.

If a woman is thinking of giving birth at home, she can discuss this with her GP, a community midwife, and independent midwife, the NCT or a local home birth support group (the local NCT branch should have details). Some GPs are very supportive of home birth and themselves attend women in labour at home or provide 'cover' for community mid-wives. Other GPs, unfortunately, are still striking women and their families off their lists for requesting a home birth although this is against government policy.[4] If a woman is unable to arrange a home birth through her GP, she can contact the local community midwives direct or telephone or write to the director of maternity services or the super-visor of midwives (sometimes these are the same person) requesting a home birth. The supervisor of midwives has a legal duty to arrange midwifery care for a woman she knows is pregnant, and this must be provided at home if that is what the women wishes (Midwives' Rules). If a GP goes so far as to strike a woman off his/her list for requesting a home birth, the woman can complain in writing to the local Family Health Services Authority (address in telephone directory).

> When I told my GP I wanted a home birth and that I didn't want him to be involved in my antenatal/delivery/postnatal care, that I only wanted to be attended by the community midwives' team, he struck me off along with my 3 year old daughter who was ill at the time (on the day the Winterton Report was published!).[5]

Many women who go ahead and book a home birth with community midwives are asked to go and see a consultant obstetrician in hospital. In most cases, this is more or less a courtesy visit, giving the woman and the obstetrician the opportunity to meet and to discuss the emergency back-up available from the hospital and the circumstances in which transfer to hospital might be advisable. In other cases, the appointment

....

4 Maternity Services, 1992.
5 National Childbirth Trust, 1992.

is used by the obstetrician to try to dissuade the woman from giving birth at home by 'shroud waving' and other unfair means. A woman invited to meet an obstetrician can usually discover from discreet enquiries what form the consultation is likely to take and may accept or decline the invitation accordingly. She does not have to go if she does not wish to. It is generally accepted that a woman should have at least one medical examination during her pregnancy to check her heart and lungs, but this can usually be done by her GP if she prefers.

THE 'BOOKING APPOINTMENT'

Once the woman has decided on her maternity care package, she will be given a 'booking appointment'. This is usually with a midwife, although in some hospitals doctors still see women for this first appointment to take a history and give a medical examination. A full medical history will be taken and the woman will be informed about the pattern of her antenatal care. The booking appointment takes place either at home, at a community clinic or at the maternity unit of her choice. There is a current trend even for women planning hospital births to have their booking appointment at home, the idea being that a woman will feel more at ease on her own territory and that there will be a more equal exchange of information between the woman and the midwife. For some women who have booked their care without the benefit of full information about the options available, the home booking appointment gives an opportunity to fill in the gaps and they may find that they wish to change their care. In fact, a woman can change her care at any time during her pregnancy, provided that the alternative system is not fully booked. Home births are not limited in this way, because, as stated above, women have a legal right to have their babies at home and midwives have a legal duty to attend them there. However, some health professionals feel that a substantial increase in the demand for home births or dominos may put undue pressure on community midwives unless resources are shifted from hospitals into the community.

GETTING THE MOST OUT OF ANTENATAL CARE

Ideally the woman will be able to get to know the midwives who will be caring for her during labour and postnatally during her antenatal care, even if some of this is shared with a GP. If a woman has booked a home birth with NHS community midwives or an independent midwife, she will probably receive most of her care at home from a team of no more than four midwives, with one midwife being 'her' midwife, taking the lead in her care and, hopefully, being the one to deliver her. Equally with a domino, GP or midwife unit package, the team of carers should be small enough for the woman to build up a relationship with them and for her caregivers to get to know the woman. The likely result is that the woman's state of health and her preferences become well-known to the team so that they are able to give her appropriate care during labour. The woman for her part feels relaxed and comfortable with people she knows so that tension is less likely to interfere with the course of her labour.

Whichever package of care a woman has chosen, it is vital that she asks questions about any part of her care which has not been explained or which she does not understand. If she has any problems at home which may affect her physical or emotional health, she should feel able to share these and to ask for professional help or support if she feels she needs it. If complications arise and she needs medical care, but does not understand what the doctor has told her or is too anxious to take it in, she can ask a midwife to give her an explanation when she feels calmer.

ANTENATAL CLASSES The uptake of antenatal classes can be low and their quality variable. But when they are good, they can be an excellent source of practical information for coping with labour and life with a new baby. They also give women and couples the opportunity to meet other people having babies at the same time and to give each other peer support which can continue after the birth. Accessibility for women who do not speak or understand English or who have physical disabilities can be a problem, as can classes held only in the daytime if women and their labour companions are at work and cannot get time off.

NHS classes are held, free of charge, both in hospitals and in community clinics. Increasingly, often in response to demand from men to be involved in antenatal classes, NHS classes are being held in the evenings and are very popular. NHS classes are usually taught by hospital or community midwives, with some input from obstetric physiotherapists and health visitors. Some hospitals arrange talks by doctors on topics such as pain relief. Every woman receiving NHS care should be offered antenatal classes and, if she wishes to attend, she should ensure a place is booked for her and, if appropriate, her labour companion.

Private classes are available, for a fee, with: the NCT; active birth teachers; some independent midwives as part of their package of care; some private maternity units for their clients; and independent childbirth educators including teachers of yoga and Alexander technique for pregnant women. Women often find out about private classes from friends or by contacting the NCT which sometimes has information about classes available with other teachers too, particularly if NCT classes become full very quickly. Any woman wanting NCT classes should contact her local branch at about twelve weeks of pregnancy to book them, because there are often not enough classes to meet demand (although in some rural areas classes can be difficult to get to and therefore there is not the same pressure on places). This can be difficult for women undergoing screening for fetal abnormality, but NCT teachers are trained to handle this issue sensitively.

What is covered in antenatal classes varies enormously. Some private classes such as active birth, yoga and Alexander technique concentrate mostly on physical ways of coping with labour and these can be all that a woman having her second or subsequent baby needs. The emphasis on the natural process of labour and encouraging women to develop awareness of their bodies and their ability to relax, breathe well and cope with pain, is useful for women intending to have as natural a birth as possible and to rely on their own resources for coping with pain. Teachers of these classes usually arrange occasional evening classes when labour companions can be shown how to support women using this kind of approach.

NHS and NCT classes usually have a balance of information about what to expect at the end of pregnancy, during labour and from life with a new baby; information about different methods of pain relief, hospital procedures and complications; a selection of relaxation, breathing and massage techniques for coping with labour; and opportunities for general discussion and questions. Because NCT classes are private, class sizes are smaller (an NCT teacher can only teach twelve women or eight couples in one class) and therefore it is easier for class members to get to know each other and to ask questions about the issues important to them. In addition, as NCT teachers are independent of the NHS and women attending their classes might have booked different packages of maternity care, discussion about the management of labour and procedures used in different settings often shows up the wide range of possibilities and enables women to have a better idea of their preferences for care. (It has been known for women to change their care as a result of discussion in NCT classes!)

Classes which teach self-help coping techniques for labour and develop a woman's confidence in her ability to give birth and in her labour companion to give support, can be very helpful. Discussing different procedures and interventions, including how to use artificial methods of pain relief well, can help a woman become aware of the sorts of things she would like to choose during her labour and those she would rather avoid.

CHOOSING A LABOUR COMPANION

As a result of campaigning by the NCT and other organisations in the 1960s, it is now generally accepted in Britain and often expected that the woman has with her in labour the father of her baby. Women often find the support of their partner invaluable during the birth and sometimes says things like 'I couldn't have done it without him.'

However, some women do not have a partner and other women are unable or unwilling to have their partner with them during labour. Equally, there are some men who do not wish to be present. In this situation, some women are happy to rely on the support of their midwives. But others find that, however sensitive and caring their midwives are, it makes a positive difference to their experience to be accompanied by someone who is not present in a professional capacity, but who is there as their friend. Some women choose to have more than one labour companion, or perhaps they invite a sister or friend in addition to their partner.

The role of the labour companion will vary according to the woman's needs, but they will usually give physical as well as moral support and sometimes repeat information given to the woman by her caregivers which she was unable to take in. If a woman wishes to avoid unnecessary interventions, her labour companion can back her up. It is important for the woman's labour companion to be involved in any antenatal preparation, especially if the woman intends to use self-help coping techniques. In this way they can support the women with knowledge of what to do as well as sensitivity to her needs.

If the woman does not speak or understand English, her midwife should be able to arrange for an interpreter or linkworker to accompany the woman during labour and at her antenatal check-ups. However, the woman may prefer a friend or relative to perform this function and should be encouraged to make her wishes known.

OTHER ANTENATAL PREPARATION

Women learn a vast amount from other women about birth. Hearing accounts of many different experiences can help a woman build up a picture of the range of possibilities in labour and give her some idea of what to expect. Although some women's birth stories may be rather negative, they can usually be balanced by positive ones. It is important for the woman to remember that her birth and her attitude to coping with it will be unique (and that therefore what worked well for another woman may not work so well for her). There is a wealth of books, magazines, leaflets and videos available for women wanting to learn more (see Further Information for Parents, page 198, for a small selection). There can often be interesting programmes on television and radio as well. All these can help a woman add to her knowledge. If she is concerned about any of the information she comes across, she can speak to her midwife or antenatal teacher who can reassure her or put it into context for her.

BIRTH PLANS

'The hospital also seemed more open to "birth plans", and asked what you wanted during the birth – which is an important aspect when having a hospital delivery.'

'What I learnt during this time was not to make too many decisions in advance but to wait until the parameters for making them were in place.'[6]

At some point during her antenatal care, perhaps during the last two or three months of her pregnancy, the woman should discuss with her midwife her preferences for labour. These could include how long she wishes to stay at home in labour before going into hospital and what sort of pain relief she may choose to use. People vary and some women write a birth plan setting out exactly what they would like to happen at every stage of their labour. Others prefer to wait and see what happens, choosing to make their decisions at the time, or are content to take the advice of the midwives and doctors looking after them during labour. The latter may be a satisfactory approach if a woman's view of birth is the same as that of her caregivers, but if the hospital's approach is very 'high-tech' and the woman would prefer a 'low-tech' approach, for example, she may have a disappointing experience. Also, if a woman has strong feelings about what she would or would not like from her care, these may get lost if they are not written down.

Currently some people have doubts about the value of birth plans. Some health professionals have been scathing about what they perceive as unrealistic, aggressively phrased birth plans insisting on no intervention, whose authors have ended up experiencing a large number of interventions, often after a change of heart. Some hospitals have short-circuited the system by producing their own form of birth plan with check-lists which may or may not correspond with an individual woman's agenda, only to ignore the plan when a woman goes into

6 National Childbirth Trust, 1992.

labour. 'At least 59% of the respondents to the *Good Housekeeping* survey had made a birth plan. For 35% the birth plan was adhered to; for 13% it was changed because of a medical emergency; 6% changed their minds; and for 4% the staff were unsupportive'.[7]

As a result, some NCT antenatal teachers are asked by their clients whether or not it is necessary to write a birth plan, as though it were somehow expected of the sort of person who attends antenatal classes outside the NHS system. The answer is that a woman should feel able to write a birth plan if she wishes but need not feel obliged to do so. In any case a woman should discuss the sort of care she would like during labour with her midwife antenatally. She may ask her partner or other labour companion to attend the appointment with her so that they are able to be present at the discussion and understand the hospital's approach to the management of labour. Alternatively (this tends to happen when a woman receives care from a small team of midwives or from an independent midwife) the woman may prefer to discuss different aspects of labour at different times during her pregnancy as her knowledge of what to expect and ideas for her own preferences develop. Another approach is for the woman and her partner each to write their own birth plans and then to compare notes.

A formal birth plan written by the woman can set the agenda for discussion with her midwife. An alternative approach is for the woman to ask about hospital policies regarding the areas of concern to her and to focus in her birth plan on those issues where her own preferences differ from hospital policy. For example, there may be a policy that every woman in labour has her waters broken by the midwife at 3 cm dilatation or on admission into hospital, whichever is the earlier. In these circumstances, the woman might ask that her waters be left to break spontaneously on the grounds that research shows that there is little benefit in breaking them early on in a normal labour. When adopting this approach, and finding that her preferences differ from hospital policy in only a few aspects, the woman may ask the midwife to record her preferences in her notes, rather than write a formal birth plan or fill in a checklist. If a woman does write a birth plan, it is advisable for it to be tactfully phased and to take account of any professional advice about the possibilities for her birth.

With a view to avoiding an unnecessary caesarean, the woman experiencing a normal pregnancy and anticipating a normal labour might choose to consider some of the following aspects of care:

7 Lewison, 1991, p. 125.

• If she is found to be in the latent phase of labour when she comes into hospital, whether she can return home until the contractions become stronger.

• Whether there is a policy for listening to the baby's heartbeat using continuous electronic fetal heart monitoring, in both normal and abnormal labour.

• Whether fetal blood sampling is used to check if abnormalities in the recording of the baby's heart rate are noted.

• Whether the waters are routinely broken artificially and if so, when, or whether they are allowed to break spontaneously.

• Whether she can eat and drink if she is hungry and thirsty throughout labour.

• Whether she can take up whichever position she feels most comfortable in at every stage of labour, even if the baby's heart is being monitored.

• Whether any time limits are set for the first and second stages of labour.

• How the onset of the active phase of labour is defined, for example, when the cervix is 3 cm dilated, fully effaced and the woman is experiencing strong regular contractions.

• In what circumstances an oxytocin drip is used to accelerate labour.

• Whether, in the latent phase of the second stage of labour, the woman is allowed to wait until she has an urge to push.

• The availability of epidural or spinal anaesthesia for an emergency caesarean.

If the woman is experiencing any complications she might in addition ask about the following:

• What effect, if any, a pre-existing medical condition or disability might have on the management of her labour.

• What effect a pregnancy-related illness such as gestational diabetes, raised blood pressure or pre-eclampsia might have on the management of her labour.

• Whether external cephalic version is attempted to turn breech babies and if so, when.

• The management of a breech labour.

• The management of a multiple birth.

• The availability of epidural or spinal anaesthesia for an elective or emergency caesarean.

• Whether her labour companion can be present during all procedures.

If a woman has written a formal birth plan, once the final form has been agreed she should prepare two copies – one for herself and one to be kept with her notes – both of which should be signed by herself and her midwife or obstetrician. In some hospitals, a woman wishing to use a birth plan is asked to see a doctor. If this is the case, the woman should insist that the doctor is not a trainee (senior house officer), but either her consultant or a senior member of his or her team whose participation in the process of negotiating the birth plan will be meaningful.

CHOOSING BETWEEN AN ELECTIVE CAESAREAN AND A TRIAL OF LABOUR

If a woman is faced with one of the relative indications for caesarean such as suspected feto-pelvic disproportion, she may be given a choice between an elective caesarean and a trial of labour. The woman will obviously discuss her choice with her obstetrician. Although the obstetrician is likely to advise her to take one course or the other, she should feel able to choose which feels right for her and, if necessary, to ask for a second opinion from another obstetrician. She should obtain as much information as there is about her obstetric condition, including the chances of delivering vaginally. She should also ask whether an epidural or spinal anaesthetic will be available to her for an elective or emergency caesarean. *'I desperately needed an epidural but the man who does these only comes in during the day!'*[8]

Some women prefer the certainty of preparing for an elective caesarean, hopefully under epidural, knowing the date on which their baby will be born and being able to make all necessary preparations, to the uncertainty of waiting for labour to begin spontaneously and then perhaps ending up with a caesarean, possibly under general anaesthetic. However, obstetricians are unlikely to offer an elective caesarean unless there is a medical reason for it. Other women prefer to give their bodies every chance to give birth unaided and, if an emergency caesarean is necessary, derive satisfaction from the knowledge that they tried everything they could to avoid a caesarean.

In a prospective study, women were asked: 'If your consultant told you that there was *a 50:50 chance* of needing a caesarean section, what would you prefer to do?' Seventeen per cent expressed a preference for caesarean section, 68 per cent for a trial of labour; 4 per cent said they would not mind; and 10 per cent that they did not know.[9] Thus the

....

8 National Childbirth Trust, 1992.
9 Green et al., 1988, pp. 6.9–10.

majority of women preferred the idea of a vaginal delivery.

It is vital that the woman presented with such a choice thinks carefully about her decision. She may find it helpful to discuss the matter with her midwife, her partner or with a woman who has gone through a similar experience (some NCT branches run caesarean support groups) as well as her obstetrician. She can then make an informed choice based on what feels right for her.

'I felt a lot of pressure to conform to the hospital policy and had to be very assertive to achieve a vaginal delivery.'[10]

'My daughter presented breech . . . I arrived at hospital 7½ cm dilated and tried to convince the consultant I wanted to deliver normally . . . He "talked me round" into having a section. In a way I feel cheated because I wasn't fully in control of myself and I was talked round.'[11]

COPING WITH A NORMAL LABOUR OR A TRIAL OF LABOUR

The same conditions apply to both if the woman is to avoid an unnecessary caesarean. In fact, the nearer the management of a trial of labour is to that of a normal labour, the more likely a woman is to be able to give birth vaginally. Ways in which a woman can be helped to deliver vaginally are as follows:

- Resisting induction of labour for non-urgent reasons if the cervix is unripe.
- Staying at home as long as possible. The woman may find that using a TENS machine or warm bath for pain relief at home enables her to delay going into hospital.
- Having a home assessment in labour from community midwives is usually possible on a domino or integrated team midwifery scheme. The woman will probably find it reassuring to be given a vaginal examination to see how far her cervix has dilated and to have the baby's heart rate checked.
- If a home assessment in labour is not possible, the woman may find it reassuring to keep in touch by telephone with midwives on the hospital labour ward who will tell her whether it is advisable to remain at home.
- Being looked after by midwives she has got to know antenatally and who know her and her preferences.

....
10 National Childbirth Trust, 1992.
11 National Childbirth Trust, 1992.

• Procedures or interventions should not be carried out for routine reasons, but because they are necessary in the woman's labour. All procedures and interventions should be explained fully to the woman, together with the reasons for performing them.

• Not being continuously connected to an electronic fetal heart rate monitor unless there is some doubt about the baby's condition. Research shows that listening to the baby's heart rate at regular intervals is just as effective. What matters is that any doubtful results should be considered carefully and any necessary action taken quickly.[12]

• Doubtful traces from the electronic fetal heart rate monitor should be checked using fetal blood sampling for further evidence of the baby's condition.

• Not having the waters broken artificially unless there is a good reason for doing so. Routine policy is an inadequate reason.

• Not having the labour accelerated using an oxytocin drip unless there is a good reason for doing so, since some babies become distressed as a result of their oxygen supply being reduced by the artificially strengthened contractions. Conforming to arbitrary time limits is an inadequate reason for acceleration unless there is a full active management of labour policy incorporating accurate diagnosis of the active phase of labour (page 57), although cessation of dilatation would be a good reason for it.

• Careful use of epidurals for routine pain relief. The woman's contractions may become weaker as a result of reduced mobility and she may then be given an oxytocin drip to strengthen the contractions, which may adversely affect the baby. Sometimes a woman undergoing a trial of labour is recommended to have an epidural so that she can be awake in the event of an emergency caesarean becoming necessary. However, managing labour in this way could make a caesarean a self-fulfilling prophecy. A woman might be much more likely to deliver vaginally if she is able to use self-help techniques such as upright position and movement to promote the natural progress of labour and to maximise the ability of her pelvis to expand to accommodate the baby. (A few hospitals are beginning to develop a 'mobile' epidural which gives pain relief without affecting the woman's mobility. This new technique has not yet been evaluated in a formal research study.)

• Being as relaxed as possible, both during and between contractions, so as not to interfere with the natural process of labour.

• She is likely to find upright positions the most comfortable and these use gravity to aid the process of labour.

....

12 MacDonald et al., 1985.

• Using a breathing technique for coping with contractions learned ante-natally. One technique is to concentrate on the outbreath, letting the breaths in take care of themselves. This ensures that the woman, the baby and the uterus have enough oxygen to cope with the hard work of labour.

• Remaining mobile and changing position. Different positions will feel comfortable at different times in labour. If the woman listens to her body she will automatically take up the position most useful for labour. If the baby is in an awkward position, walking around, pelvic rocking and other rhythmic movements may help it to turn into the right position.

• Touch and massage. Good for contractions experienced as back pain and for helping the woman feel less isolated during contractions. If the woman finds that she does not want to be touched or held in labour, she should make this known to those with her!

• Darkness promotes the release of endorphins, the body's natural pain-killers produced in response to pain. Another way of helping the woman concentrate on herself and her labour if she wears glasses or contact lenses is to remove them. But the woman may prefer to keep them on and may also appreciate eye contact to help her stay with the contractions.

• Food and drink. Essential during a long labour since a labouring woman uses 700–1,000 calories per hour. Many hospitals do not allow even women at low risk of complications to eat or drink during the active phase of labour on the grounds that they may inhale acid stomach contents during a general anaesthetic. However, research shows that it is usually faulty anaesthetic technique and insufficiently experienced operators which cause this to happen. Possible ways round such a policy are to put unrestricted eating and drinking in a birth plan, to stay at home as long as possible and to eat and drink right up to the end of the latent phase of labour. However, do eat easily digestible food.

• Using large cushions, beanbags, birthing chairs, music, etc. to get as comfortable as possible. A labour companion is good to lean on too!

• Using a birthing pool or warm bath can be an effective form of pain relief and may help the woman stay relaxed, particularly if she uses long baths as a way of coping with everyday life. However, the use of water for pain relief in labour has not been scientifically evaluated.

• Natural therapies such as homoeopathy, acupuncture, hypnotherapy, aromatherapy, etc. can be useful in labour if the woman uses them in her normal life and if she knows a practitioner who will attend her in labour. The advantage of hypnotherapy is that the woman is usually taught self-hypnosis for labour so that the practitioner does not have to be on call. Some homoeopaths suggest a kit of remedies useful for labour and instruct the woman (and her labour companion) when to use them in labour or suggest remedies over the telephone. Supporters of natural therapies believe that they can promote the normal progress of labour and thus keep interventions to a minimum.

HOW ANTENATAL TEACHERS CAN HELP

It is clear from our study of women's experiences that they require more information about caesareans. This includes what to expect both during and after the procedure and the implications of being awake or asleep for the operation. All antenatal classes should incorporate this information as well as caesarean statistics. Thus women might realise that the experience is not so rare as one would hope and that there are choices they can make both to reduce the risk of a caesarean occurring and to make the experience, if it happens to them, as well as its aftermath, as positive as possible.

At the same time, the most valuable role of the antenatal teacher is to instil in women the confidence that they can probably give birth vaginally and that there are many choices women can make to increase the likelihood of a vaginal delivery, provided that labour progresses normally. Although the current caesarean rate is high, nevertheless antenatal teachers can put this figure into perspective, particularly if they have access to up-to-date caesarean rates for local hospitals, and can remind women that the overwhelming chances are that they will not have a caesarean delivery. Over 95 per cent of women who start labour naturally at term should deliver vaginally.

HOW GPs CAN HELP

We believe that unless the GP is prepared to give the whole package of maternity care, including intrapartum care, or cover during labour for midwives attending women at home or in GP maternity units, the role of the GP should be limited to providing emotional support to the woman and her family and continuing medical care.[13] It is therefore vital that GPs give women full information about the local options for maternity care, including arrangements for obtaining a home birth if this is a service that the GP does not offer.[14] Sometimes, making their premises available to midwives and obstetricians wishing to take antenatal care into the community in order to make it more accessible to women may also help facilitate continuity of carer and may make GPs more confident.

....

13 NHS Management Executive, 1993.
14 Maternity Services, 1992.

HOW MIDWIVES CAN HELP

Midwives are generally acknowledged as the experts in normal childbirth and are trained to identify when pregnancy and birth become abnormal. It is part of their professional duty to refer women for appropriate medical assistance. Therefore midwives should expect to give women an increasing proportion of their care, so that obstetricians can use their skills for the benefit of women experiencing complications. Changes are currently being made in maternity care all over Britain to devise local schemes enabling smaller teams of midwives to look after identified caseloads of women throughout their pregnancy, birth and the postnatal period. When a woman ends up needing medical assistance, the fact that she continues to receive support from midwives known to her is likely to make her experience a positive one. Therefore we encourage midwives to rise to the challenge of working in new and flexible ways so as to increase both women's satisfaction and their own.

On an individual level, midwives can try to make every encounter with a woman meaningful; to ensure that the woman understands the purpose and outcome of the meeting; and that she goes away having been able to ask questions and have them answered to her satisfaction. On an organisational level, midwives can set up a midwifery practice group in their maternity unit or district to support each other in times of change; to examine their practice; and to aim at achieving improvements in the service they offer to women. These improvements should include more continuity of carer and would, we hope, lower caesarean section rates where these are high.

HOW OBSTETRICIANS CAN HELP

We invite obstetricians to look critically at caesarean rates in their unit and at their own practice. Could their team's caesarean rate be lowered? How does it compare with the rates of other teams, and with the current national rate we have found of 13 per cent? Are they performing unnecessary caesareans? Could maternity care be organised differently so that women experiencing normal pregnancies and births were cared for entirely by midwives? This would give obstetricians more time to look at each woman experiencing complications individually and to advise care, taking into account her needs rather than under a blanket policy.

Before operating, the consultant examined me vaginally and found me sufficiently dilated to see that the placenta was not in the way and also he managed to turn the baby's head down. I was therefore allowed to 'come round' [from the general anaesthetic] and delivered vaginally two hours later . . . he felt it right to 'let me have a go myself' in view of the problems recovering from a section would have caused my family . . . I felt that this was a brave decision – many consultants faced with an unconscious patient and a theatre full of staff would have carried on![15]

A US study carried out in a teaching hospital serving 'a largely high-risk, low-income obstetric population' describes how the caesarean section rate declined from 27.5 per cent in 1986 to 10.5 per cent in 1989.[16] A larger proportion of women attempted a trial of labour after repeat caesarean (a rise from 32 to 84 per cent); more women having a trial of labour gave birth vaginally (a rise from 65 to 83 per cent); there were fewer caesareans for dystocia and fetal distress (a fall from 14 to 4 per cent of all deliveries). This was achieved without increasing perinatal mortality rates. The methods used were introduced on 1 July 1987 and were as follows:

● New guidelines for the management of labour for women with previous caesarean sections.
● New guidelines for performing caesareans on first-time mothers, taking into account dystocia, fetal distress and fetal malposition.
● Weekly conferences at which medical staff reviewed the reasons for which each caesarean section had been performed.

The study concluded:

Our success in lowering cesarean section rates is largely attributable to our centralized approach to intrapartum decision making . . . it contrasts with other approaches many obstetric units in this country use, in which cesarean section rates for individual obstetricians may vary markedly . . . Implementing standardized protocols . . . requires substantial commitment and effort from obstetricians and others who care for obstetric patients. However, our experience suggests that such an effort can substantially reduce rates of cesarean delivery without compromising the newborn.[17]

....
15 National Childbirth Trust, 1992.
16 Sanchez-Ramos et al., 1990.
17 Sanchez-Ramos et al., 1990, p. 1086.

Similar efforts have been made in Canada,[18] Glasgow and Manchester, where individual obstetricians have taken the lead in reducing the caesarean rate by encouraging peers to examine the reasons for performing caesareans. We would therefore encourage more obstetricians to consider taking on this role.

Three specific measures are as follows. Induction of labour should be a consultant decision. The use of the fax machine to fax CTG traces and partograms to keep the duty consultant up to date about the labour ward should improve decision making.[19] Leaving women with ruptured membranes to go into labour spontaneously has also been shown to reduce the caesarean rate.[20]

It is also time for the Royal College of Obstetricians and Gynaecologists (RCOG) to examine the caesarean section rates and their wide variation between maternity units and to consider what can be done to reduce the ones that are obviously too high. One of the problems has been that the latest figures published by the government are those for 1985, when the rate was 10.5 per cent. Now that our sample has indicated a probable rate of 13 per cent for 1992, we hope that the RCOG will be moved to set up a study group to examine the issue, publish a report and make recommendations for improvements in practice.

The training of obstetricians was an issue brought to our attention by the consultants in our survey and we support the recent initiative by the RCOG to make improvements. In this connection, we would also support the recommendations of the House of Commons Health Committee's 1992 report which said that junior doctors should work in a supernumerary capacity and receive adequate supervision in order to acquire training of a suitable standard.[21]

The issue of performing caesareans for medico-legal reasons rather than clinical reasons is one which needs to be dealt with as a matter of urgency. Lawyers as well as obstetricians need to take account of the research evidence and to look critically at some of the legal judgements which have been made.[22] Our sample of consultant obstetricians showed a very positive interest in some system of no-fault compensation for all babies born handicapped and this issue needs urgent consideration. However, two recent British documents and experience outside Britain

....

18 Lomas, 1991.
19 Quinn, 1993.
20 Hofmeyr and Keirse, 1990.
21 Health Committee, 1992, para. 364.
22 Giesen, 1993.

suggest that no-fault compensation may not necessarily be the best solution.[23]

One underlying problem is the way that medicine is portrayed by the media – encouraged by some doctors. It appears to be 'cut and dried' but much of what doctors do, obstetricians included, is not based on hard evidence. There is not always a correct way to help a woman in labour. If, as may happen in at least one pregnancy in 600, the baby dies for reasons which nobody understands, the obstetrician is sued for not doing more and this increases the risk of women having unnecessary caesareans.

HOW MATERNITY UNITS CAN HELP

The providers of maternity care can help by publishing their caesarean and other intervention rates annually. The annual report of St George's Hospital, London, is an admirable example of an informative document written in an accessible, self-critical manner.[24] If possible, rates should also be given for each individual consultant. If particular consultants specialise in caring for women with a high risk of caesarean section, this could be explained.

The maternity booklets given by every maternity unit to women should contain meaningful information about hospital policies for routine procedures and interventions for complications, options for anaesthesia during caesareans, and up-to-date intervention rates. Women using the service would be better informed and might be empowered to express their needs more effectively than is often possible at present. Establishing schemes whereby continuity of carer can be achieved would also facilitate this process. All written information for women should be accessible in other relevant languages for the community as well as in braille. Videos and audiotapes should also be available where appropriate.

Every provider unit should be auditing every aspect of its clinical care, including caesarean rates and women's satisfaction with their care. The results of this audit should be used to refine practice and reduce the number of unnecessary caesareans. It is hoped that the advent of clinical directorates will assist in this process.

HOW PURCHASING AUTHORITIES CAN HELP

One of the roles of district health authorities when purchasing maternity care is to set quality standards. They then

....

23 ACHCEW, 1992; Spastics Society, 1992.
24 Chamberlain and Peattie, 1991.

negotiate with different providers to what level each standard should apply, the aim being that all the providers in a district will eventually meet the same standards for each category of care. Standards should therefore be set, aimed at minimising the number of unnecessary caesareans, since these are an unnecessary drain on resources.

HOW MATERNITY SERVICES LIAISON COMMITTEES (MSLCs) CAN HELP

MSLCs exist in many district health authorities as forums where representatives from all the relevant professional groups as well as maternity services managers meet together with consumer representatives to consider maternity services and to advise both purchasing authorities and provider units. The 1992 Health Committee report made a number of recommendations designed to make them work more effectively and also recommended particular issues on which they could advise at local level.[25] It is suggested that the question of unnecessary caesareans is a suitable issue for MSLCs to tackle. In addition, MSLCs are well placed to assist GPs, midwives and obstetricians as well as purchasing authorities and provider units in working together to avoid unnecessary caesareans.

HOW READERS OF THIS BOOK CAN HELP

If you care about the rise in unnecessary caesareans, you may use the information in this book to make changes at local level to reduce their number. You may be a woman who hopes to avoid a first delivery by caesarean, or a repeat caesarean; a midwife newly promoted to a management position; an antenatal teacher asked to sit on an MSLC; or an obstetrician concerned enough about the issue to read this book. All of you have a role to play in keeping caesareans to the minimum necessary for the safety of women and their babies and in preventing unnecessary caesareans from blighting the first few weeks of a mother and baby's relationship.

....

25 Health Committee, 1992, paras 445, 218 and 243.

APPENDICES

SIX TYPES OF CARE FOR BIRTH

The table below is based on NCT leaflets prepared to explain to women the main features of the different packages of maternity care on offer in Britain. At first sight, the table may seem complex, but it is not nearly as

Package of care	Who gives antenatal care?	Where is antenatal care given?	Place of birth
Home birth	Community or independent midwives and/or GP	At home or in GP surgery or community clinic	At home
Total hospital care	Hospital midwives and doctors	Hospital antenatal clinic	Hospital
'Shared care'	GP, often assisted by community midwife, and hospital midwives and doctors	GP surgery and hospital antenatal clinic	Hospital
Domino scheme	Community midwives (can be combined with shared care from GP)	At home or GP surgery or midwives' clinic in community or in hospital	Hospital
Integrated midwifery scheme	Small team of midwives working in hospital and in the community	At home or midwives' clinic in community or in hospital	At home or in hospital
GP- or midwife-led unit delivery	GP and community midwives	GP surgery or at home or midwives' clinic in community or in unit	Isolated unit or unit alongside district general hospital

complicated as the system which it aims to explain! By choosing one of the packages of care in the first column on the left, you can discover the main features by reading horizontally across to the right. If you are particularly interested in one feature of care such as giving birth at home, for example, you can choose the column entitled 'Place of birth' and read down vertically to see which packages of care offer this option.

Who delivers the baby?	Essential features of the package	With whom to book your care
Community or independent midwife with cover from GP or hospital	All your care takes place at home and you have the chance to get to know the midwife or small team of midwives, one of whom will attend your birth	Community midwives or GP or via supervisor of midwives
Hospital midwife. In a teaching hospital a student midwife or doctor under supervision. Cover from obstetricians	All care conducted by hospital-based midwives and doctors directly responsible to consultant obstetricians whose (individual) policies will determine the way care is provided	GP or direct with the hospital: ring and ask for the antenatal clinic
As above	Similar to a hospital birth except that many routine antenatal appointments are with your GP or community midwives. Many women welcome this more personal form of care which may mean less travel and shorter waiting times	Your GP or, if s/he does not offer the service, or if you prefer, with another GP
Community midwife. Cover from obstetricians	All care is given by a community midwife or small team of community midwives, so you get to know the person who will attend your delivery, provided there are flexible working patterns. An important bonus is that a community midwife assesses you in labour at home. 6-hour discharge if you want.	Your GP or with the community midwives: ring them at your local maternity unit
Team midwife. Cover as above	You receive individualised care from a small team you get to know well	The team via your GP or the local hospital
GP or community midwives. Cover from GP or district general hospital	A personal form of care popular in rural areas with a high rate of continuity of carer	Your GP or another GP or with the community midwives

METHODOLOGY OF THE TWO SURVEYS

SURVEY OF WOMEN'S EXPERIENCES (CHAPTER 7)

This study utilised a survey designed to assess the experiences of women having caesarean sections. The aims of the survey were: first, to find out from women the reasons they had been given for their operations in order that a comparison could be made with the reasons given by consultants; second, to analyse women's experiences of caesarean birth in the light of current debate on medical intervention and to suggest ways in which the management of birth can best be achieved for all concerned.

The Sampling Procedure

A sample consisting of one hospital from each of the fourteen regions was randomly selected. Permission to conduct the survey of women's experiences was requested from consultant obstetricians responsible in each case. Eleven hospitals, geographically spread across the country, agreed to take part in the study. The two-page questionnaires were sent out along with covering letters to the participating hospitals with the request that they be handed to fifty consecutive women having caesareans.

The Questionnaire

The questionnaire asked for quantitative data about the women, the operations and the babies, as well as qualitative information regarding the women's experiences and feelings about the births. The questionnaires were coded and entered onto a computer where the data were analysed using the Supastats package.

The Response Rate

Completed questionnaires were received from nine of the eleven participating hospitals, i.e. a response rate of 81.8 per cent. Information provided by the hospitals revealed that over 90 per cent of the women invited to help with the study completed a questionnaire. The first 300 questionnaires received are analysed here. Of these, 132 (44 per cent) were elective caesareans and 168 (56 per cent) were emergency operations. The women were further divided into three categories: first births, previous vaginal deliveries and previous deliveries including caesareans.

The data show that almost half (47.3 per cent) of caesarean sections are being carried out on women who are giving birth for the first time. Furthermore the majority of those women (68.5 per cent) are having emergency operations. Three out of five (60.6 per cent) women having elective sections have had previous caesareans.

METHODOLOGY OF THE CONSULTANTS SURVEY (CHAPTER 8)

Using the 1989 *Medical Directory*, we set out to draw a random sample of approximately 50 per cent of the consultants in England and Wales, stratified to ensure that one consultant was drawn from each hospital. We began with a sample of 404 in England and 26 in Wales. All of the obstetricians in Scotland (127) were surveyed as their views had not been obtained in the earlier studies. A two-page questionnaire was sent out on 13 February 1990; second and third mailings were sent on 23 May and 10 August 1990 to those who did not respond. In September and October 1990 we phoned those who had not replied. After data entry and preliminary analysis, some consultants were asked to clarify their responses in February 1991. The questionnaires were analysed using the SPSS package. An article based on these results was published by Savage and Francome in the *Journal of Obstetrics and Gynaecology* in May 1993. However, once the decision to write a book had been taken, Colin Francome wrote to 110 consultants who had not replied with an abbreviated questionnaire on 22 October 1992.

We looked at the response rate by hospital. According to the RCOG manpower survey in 1989 there were 228 hospitals performing obstetrics and gynaecology in England and Wales during this year. We had data from at least 68 per cent of hospitals, and some from which we did not obtain data closed or stopped doing obstetrics. In Scotland we had data for 20 of the 24 hospitals we had surveyed, giving an 83 per cent response rate.

We received 352 completed questionnaires, giving us a 71 per cent response rate from the consultants. Not every question was answered by each consultant, so in the later tables we have given the number who responded to each one. In all, 19 (3 per cent) consultants refused to reply. Another 20 consultants had either retired or were doing gynaecology only. To calculate the caesarean rate, we allowed for home deliveries and GP units.

TABLES

Table A1 *Reasons for caesarean sections*

	Elective		Emergency		Total	
	No.	%	No.	%	No.	%
I had a previous caesarean	75	56.8	12	7.1	87	29.0
Baby too big for my pelvis	55	41.7	31	18.5	86	28.7
Labour taking a long time	3	2.3	71	42.3	74	24.7
Baby was distressed (fetal distress)	1	0.8	61	36.3	62	20.7
Baby in breech position	38	28.8	19	11.3	57	19.0
Bleeding before birth	4	3.0	12	7.1	16	5.3
Cord around baby's neck	2	1.5	11	6.5	13	4.3
Baby lying across womb (transverse)	4	3.0	5	3.0	9	3.0
Baby was small for dates	4	3.0	3	1.8	7	2.3
I had diabetes	4	3.0	2	1.2	6	2.0
Cord prolapse	1	0.8	2	1.2	3	1.0
Other reasons as specified	25	18.9	40	23.8	65	21.7
Total reasons	216	269	485			
Average no. reasons per woman	1.6		1.6		1.6	
Total women	132		168		300	

Note: percentages total more than 100 as some women were given a number of reasons for their caesareans.

Table A2 *Partner's attendance at a caesarean*

	Elective		Emergency		Total	
	No.	%	No.	%	No.	%
Partner present	85	65.9	75	46.3	160	55.0
Partner not present	44	34.1	87	53.7	131	45.0
Total	129	100	162	100	291	100

Note: Women who did not answer are excluded from this table.

Table A3   *Were women adequately informed about their condition?*

	Elective		Emergency		Both groups	
	No.	%	No.	%	No.	%
Yes	125	95.4	134	81.7	259	87.8
No	6	4.6	30	18.3	36	12.2
Total	131	100	164	100	295	100

Note: Women who answered 'don't know' to this question are excluded from the table.

Table A4   *Whether women having caesareans feel that they suffer*

	Elective		Emergency		Total	
	No.	%	No.	%	No.	%
Yes	26	20.0	90	55.9	116	39.9
No	104	80.0	71	44.1	175	60.1
Total	130	100	161	100	291	100

Note: Women who did not answer are excluded from this table.

Table A5   *'Would you perform a caesarean for fetal distress to deliver a woman at a) 24 weeks or b) 26 weeks?'*

	24 weeks		26 weeks	
	No.	%	No.	%
Yes	12	3.5	100	30.5
No	261	76.3	44	13.4
Depends	69	20.2	184	56.1
Total	342	100	328	100

Table A6   *'Do you follow a policy of once a caesar, always a caesar?'*

	England and Wales		Scotland		Total UK	
	No.	%	No.	%	No.	
Yes	3	1.1	3	4.1	6	
No	272	97.8	70	95.9	342	
Did not say	3	1.1		0.0	3	
Total	278	100	73	100	351	

Table A7 *'What proportion of women with previous caeasareans had a vaginal delivery?'*

	England and Wales		Scotland	
	No.	%	No.	%
20–9%	5	3.2		
30–9%	17	10.9	3	6.7
40–9%	26	16.7	2	4.4
50–9%	47	30.1	25	55.6
60–9%	52	33.3	14	31.1
80% +	9	5.8	1	2.2
Total	156	100	45	100

Table A8   *'Do you monitor all women electronically in labour?'*

	England and Wales		Scotland		Total UK	
	No.	%	No.	%	No.	%
Yes	123	44.8	32	45.1	155	44.9
No	151	55.2	39	54.9	190	55.1
Total	274	100	71	100	345	100

Table A9   *Criteria for monitoring*

Monitor 'at risk' babies	75
Depends on mother's wishes	13
All inductions	6
Availability of machine	5
Meconium	5
Multiple births (twins)	5
Intra-uterine growth retardation	5
Fetal distress	5
Abnormality	4
If indicated as labour progresses	3
As assessed by midwives	3
Breech delivery	2
Epidural	2
Diabetes	2
Hypertension	2
Previous caesarean	2
Other reasons	11
Total	150

Table A10 *'Do you think that no-fault compensation for the parents of brain-damaged infants should be introduced?'*

	England and Wales		Scotland		All	
	No.	%	No.	%	No.	%
Yes	229	84.5	55	80.9	284	83.8
No	35	12.9	11	16.2	46	13.6
Don't know	7	2.6	2	2.9	9	2.6
Total	**271**	**100**	**68**	**100**	**339**	**100**

Table A11 *'Do you have a time limit in labour after which a caesarean is normally performed?'*

	England and Wales		Scotland		All	
	No.	%	No.	%	No.	%
No time limit	244	90.0	60	83.3	304	88.6
9 hours	3	1.1	1	1.4	4	1.2
12 hours	14	5.2	6	8.3	20	5.8
14 hours	2	0.7	0	0.0	2	0.6
16/18 hours	4	1.4	1	1.4	5	1.5
20/24 hours	3	1.1	4	5.6	7	2.0
36 hours	1	0.4	0	0.0	1	0.3
Total	**271**	**100**	**72**	**100**	**343**	**100**

Table A12 *'What proportion of caesareans are performed under epidural?'*

% caesareans under epidural	Number	%
10% or less	31	10.3
11–50%	139	46.2
51–100%	131	43.5
Total	**301**	**100**

THE LATEST BRITISH HOSPITAL DATA, 1992

Note: Hospitals with high rates may well have specialist units and so receive pregnancies which are at greater risk.

	Deliveries	Caesarean section	Rate (%)
Airedale General	2,266	270	11.9
All Saints, Kent	4,453	682	15.3
Arrowe Park, Upton, Wirral	4,260	603	14.2
Ashford, Middlesex	1,683	199	11.8
Aylesbury Vale	2,314	236	10.2
Barrat Maternity, Northampton	4,140	662	16.0
Basildon	2,489	371	14.9
Bassetlaw	1,368	170	12.4
Birch Hill, Rochdale	2,236	277	12.4
Birmingham Maternity (1991)	4,980	988	19.8
Buckland, Dover	1,089	141	12.9
Burton, Trent	3,193	418	13.1
Central Middlesex	2,104	269	12.8
Chase Farm, Enfield	3,655	469	12.8
City Maternity, Carlisle	2,134	237	11.1
Darlington Memorial	1,472	190	12.9
Dewsbury District, Yorkshire	2,836	359	12.7
Doncaster Women's	4,377	648	14.8
Dudley Road, Birmingham	4,205	531	12.6
Ealing Maternity	2,592	391	15.1
Eastbourne, Sussex	1,888	279	14.8
East Glamorgan, Pontypridd	2,129	284	13.3
East Surrey, Redhill	2,500	349	14.0
Farnborough Maternity, Orpington	3,639	452	12.4
Freedom Fields, Plymouth	5,600	672	12.0
Friarage, Northallerton	1,399	165	11.8
Frimley Park, Camberley, Surrey	2,817	333	11.8
Furness, Barrow-in-Furness	1,441	232	16.1
Good Hope, Sutton Coldfield	3,334	437	13.1
Gravesend and North Kent	3,170	493	15.6
Greenwich	3,228	437	13.5
Hammersmith	1,074	231	21.5
Harold Wood, Essex	2,343	294	12.5
Hemel Hempstead	2,746	245	9.0

	Deliveries	Caesarean section	Rate (%)
Hillingdon, nr Uxbridge	3,508	356	10.1
Homerton, London E9	3,656	612	16.7
Hope, Salford	3,103	529	17.0
Ipswich	3,309	455	13.8
Kent & Canterbury	2,218	292	13.2
Kettering General	3,497	488	14.0
Leicester General	3,982	578	14.5
Lister Maternity, Stevenage	2,976	339	11.4
Louise Margaret Maternity Wing, Aldershot	1,137	103	9.1
Marston Green, Birmingham	2,957	510	17.2
Mid-Essex (St John's)	3,914	371	9.5
Newham General, London E13	4,244	515	12.1
Norfolk & Norwich, Norwich	5,008	731	14.6
North Tees General, Stockton-on-Tees	2,427	326	13.4
Northwick Park, Harrow	3,433	457	13.3
Nuneaton Maternity	2,816	341	12.2
Pembury, nr Tunbridge Wells	2,828	318	11.2
Peterborough Maternity	3,211	461	14.4
Princess Alexandra, Harlow	3,044	407	13.4
Queen Charlotte's, London	4,043	712	17.6
Queen Mary's University, Roehampton	1,754	278	15.9
Queen's Park, Blackburn	3,734	391	10.5
Rosie Maternity, Cambridge	4,534	411	9.1
Royal Cornwall, Truro	3,156	497	15.7
Royal Hampshire, Winchester	2,534	322	12.7
Royal Lancaster	1,866	274	14.7
Royal London	3,496	405	11.6
Royal Oldham	3,399	490	14.4
Royal Shrewsbury	4,183	583	15.1
attached GP units	1,570	0	0.0
Royal Surrey, Guildford	2,816	423	15.0
Rush Green, Romford	2,445	325	13.3
Salisbury Maternity	2,149	286	13.3
Singleton, Swansea	3,512	423	12.0
Southlands, Shoreham-by-Sea	2,373	334	14.1
South Tyneside	1,980	281	14.2
Stafford District	2,553	406	15.9
St George's, London	3,339	554	16.6
St John's, Chelmsford	3,999	315	7.9
St Mary's, Isle of Wight	n.a.	n.a.	12.1
St Mary's, Portsmouth	6,641	825	12.4
St Michael's, Bristol	4,267	477	11.1
St Richard's, Chichester	2,202	265	12.0

	Deliveries	Caesarean section	Rate (%)
Tameside General, Ashton-under-Lyne	3,134	280	9.0
Taunton & Somerset	2,876	381	13.2
Torbay, Torquay	2,634	311	11.8
Warrington, Cheshire	3,332	685	20.6
West Cumberland, Whitehaven	1,630	183	11.25
Whiston, Preston, Merseyside	3,411	558	16.4
Whittington, London N19	2,809	422	15.0
William Harvey, Ashford, Kent	2,294	420	18.3
Withington, West Didsbury, Manchester	1,847	284	15.4
Worcester Royal Infirmary	2,477	511	20.6
York	3,179	472	14.8

Hospitals which gave us data but asked us to keep them confidential: Barnsley DGH, Basingstoke, Bedford, Bishop Auckland, Bronglais (Aberystwyth), Buchanan (St Leonard's-on-Sea), Dryburn (Durham), Edgware, Epsom, Gloucester Maternity, Grantham, Haelor (Clwyd), Halifax, Harrogate General, Hereford County, Hinchingbrooke, H.M. Stanley, James Paget (Gt Yarmouth), King's College, Kingston, Luton & Dunstable, Manygates (Wakefield), Mayday (Croydon), Newmarket, Northern General (Sheffield), North Manchester, North Middlesex, North Staffordshire, Nottingham City, Pontefract, Poole, Princess Royal (Hull), Queen Elizabeth (Gateshead), Queen Mary's (Sidcup, Kent), Royal Sussex (Brighton), Royal United Bath, Roy Hartley, Sharoe Green (Fulwood), Solihull, Sorrento Maternity (Moseley), Southmead (Westbury-on-Trym), St David's (Bangor), St Thomas's (London), Sunderland, Watford General, West Middlesex (Isleworth), West Suffolk (Bury St Edmunds), Westwood (Beverley) and Wycombe General.

GLOSSARY

active birth Giving birth in positions comfortable for the mother, often using gravity and not lying down on a bed.

active phase (of labour) When contractions are strong, regular and begin to open the cervix beyond 3 cm.

Alexander technique A natural therapy in which the Alexander teacher encourages the client to use the body in accordance with its natural alignment.

amniotic fluid The sterile fluid in which the baby moves and grows within the membranes.

antacids Drugs used to neutralise the stomach contents.

areola The dark-coloured area of the nipple.

assisted delivery When a mother needs help with giving birth to her baby. Usually refers to forceps, Ventouse and caesarean section.

augmentation (of labour) Speeding up labour using a synthetic oxytocin drip.

breech presentation The position of a baby who is head-up, bottom-down, before labour begins (see illustration on page 62).

cannula See *intravenous drip*.

catheter A tube inserted into the urethra to assist the passing of urine.

cauterisation Sealing blood vessels by burning to reduce bleeding.

cephalic presentation The normal position for a baby before labour begins: head-down.

cerebral palsy Brain damage occurring either before or during birth resulting in physical and, less often, in mental disability.

cerebrospinal fluid The fluid which surrounds the brain and spinal cord. This can leak out if the membrane surrounding the spinal cord is accidentally punctured during the insertion of an epidural or spinal block.

cervix The neck of the uterus. Before term it is usually long, closed and firm. As pregnancy progresses it 'ripens' and becomes soft, shorter and opens up.

classical (caesarean) section or scar A vertical cut in the upper part of the uterus.

colostrum The first milk produced by the breasts during pregnancy and for the first few days after birth. It is particularly rich in antibodies which protect the baby against infection.

Community Health Council A statutory body set up in each district health authority to represent and safeguard the interests of users of all local health services. Can help users with information and with making complaints.

community midwives Midwives working outside hospital whose work includes attending home births and domino deliveries, seeing women antenatally and postnatally, at home, in GPs' surgeries and community clinics. (See also Appendix A.)

consultant (doctor) The most senior grade of hospital doctors who have teams of junior doctors working under them and who have considerable influence on how hospitals are run. They are often involved in research and teaching and tend to see complicated rather than normal cases. Sometimes these doctors are employed by a university as lecturers, etc., rather than a health authority, and some of them have the title 'professor' rather than 'mister' or 'ms'. The majority of NHS consultants also do private work, which is why they are not employed for NHS work full-time: some consultants work in their NHS hospital for only two half-days a week, owing to their other commitments.

CTG Cardiotacograph. See *electronic fetal heart monitor*.

dehiscence The medical term for a caesarean scar coming apart, but not rupturing the uterus.

dextrose A sterile solution of sugar and water sometimes given to newborn babies in hospital. Healthy newborn babies should never be given dextrose but should be put to the breast whenever they are hungry.

dilatation (often popularly called 'dilation') The opening of the neck of the uterus (the cervix) during labour. The cervix dilates or opens to about 10 cm diameter so that the baby can be born.

dilatation and curettage ('D & C') A minor operation carried out under general anaesthetic to gently scrape the inner walls of the uterus. Performed if any pieces of placenta or membranes remain after delivery and cause heavy bleeding or infection.

disproportion See *feto-pelvic disproportion.*

domino birth See Appendix A.

dystocia The medical term for difficult labour or when a labour 'fails to progress'.

eclampsia The severe form of pre-eclampsia (see below) when a mother has fits or convulsions. It is also often associated with blood-clotting problems.

elective (caesarean) section A caesarean performed before labour has begun.

electronic fetal heart monitor A machine which collects information about a baby's heartbeat using ultrasound from a belt on the mother's abdomen or a clip fastened to the baby's head ('fetal scalp electrode'). The information is printed out continuously onto a strip of paper (a 'trace') which hospital staff can read during labour and which forms part of the permanent record of the birth.

emergency (caesarean) section A caesarean performed once labour has begun, i.e. not always in an emergency situation.

Entonox A half-and-half mixture of oxygen and nitrous oxide, inhaled for pain relief during labour.

epidural (anaesthesia) A form of local ('regional') anaesthesia used to numb the abdomen for routine pain relief during labour and total pain relief during a caesarean.

episiotomy A cut made into the perineum, using surgical scissors, to enlarge the vaginal opening before delivery. It can be performed by either a midwife or a doctor.

external cephalic version The procedure whereby an obstetrician attempts to turn a breech baby into a more favourable position before labour begins.

fetal blood sampling A medical procedure performed during labour whereby a sample of blood is taken from the baby's head and tested for acid levels as a measure of how much oxygen is being transferred to the baby.

fetal distress When the baby in the uterus is short of oxygen. It can be diagnosed by changes in the baby's heart rate and sometimes from the baby passing meconium into the amniotic fluid, as well as by fetal blood sampling.

fetal hypoxia See *fetal distress.*

feto-pelvic disproportion When the baby cannot pass through the woman's pelvis, either due to the relative size of the baby's head and the size and shape of the woman's pelvis, or because of the baby's position.

fetus The medical word for a baby before it is born.

fibroids Thickened muscle fibres in the uterine wall which are usually benign but which sometimes cause problems in pregnancy and labour.

firm The old-fashioned word for a consultant's 'team' of junior doctors and medical students.

forceps Medical instruments used by a doctor to help a woman deliver her baby. They are rather like a pair of salad servers which are inserted into the woman's vagina around the baby's head, locked together and then pulled and sometimes turned during contractions to help the baby out. They come in different sizes, depending on the sort of help the baby needs. An episiotomy is usually needed for a forceps delivery.

gestation The length of time needed for a baby to develop fully in the mother's body: this can be anything from thirty-seven to forty-two weeks.

gestational diabetes A condition whereby a woman's body does not produce enough insulin during pregnancy. Modern maternity care has made all forms of diabetes less hazardous for both mothers and babies.

glucose The fuel available in the blood for energy.

glycogen The stored form of energy which is broken down as needed to give glucose.

haemorrhage Heavy bleeding. Postpartum haemorrhage is defined as the loss of more than 500 ml of blood.

high risk A way of describing women who are more likely to experience complications or lose their babies.

hysterectomy An operation to remove the uterus.

incision The medical term for 'cut'.

induction (of labour) Starting off labour artificially using prostaglandins, breaking the membranes and, if necessary, stimulating contractions using a synthetic oxytocin drip.

instrumental delivery Giving birth with the aid of forceps or Ventouse.

integrated midwifery teams See Appendix A.

intra-uterine growth retardation (IUGR) When the baby appears not to be growing as it should. It is difficult to diagnose accurately, even using an ultrasound scan.

intravenous drip Fluid introduced into the body via a tube into a needle inserted into a vein in the arm (a 'cannula').

latent phase (of labour) The early part of labour when contractions are relatively mild, possibly irregular and have not opened the cervix beyond 3 cm.

lower-segment (caesarean) section Usually a horizontal cut in the lower part of the uterus.

Maternity Services Liaison Committee (MSLC) A committee set up by a district health authority to enable representatives from the different groups of health professionals, voluntary organisations and users to influence local policy for maternity care and to monitor the provision of services.

meconium The waste products of development retained in the baby's intestines before birth. If the baby passes meconium during labour, the amniotic fluid turns brown and this can be, but is not always, a sign of fetal distress.

membranes The tissues forming a bag around the amniotic fluid in which the baby grows in the uterus. After birth, they are usually expelled with the placenta.

midwife Usually a nurse (most are women, but a few are men) who undergoes further training in the care of women and their babies during pregnancy, labour and postnatally. In some institutions, direct-entry or 'pre-registration' training is available whereby people train solely as midwives.

morbidity The medical term for illness, disease or a physical condition other than health.

mortality The medical term for death.

multigravida (sometimes shortened to 'multip') A woman having her second or subsequent baby.

neonate Newborn baby.

no-fault compensation Awarding money to people with injuries arising from medical care, without their having to prove negligence.

obstetrician A doctor specialising in pregnancy and childbirth. A gynaecologist specialises in women's medicine and may or may not have obstetric qualifications as well.

obstetric physiotherapist See *physiotherapist*.

oedema The medical word for swelling.

ovarian cyst A growth on the ovary, usually benign, which may cause problems during labour.

oxytocin The hormone which causes the uterus to contract during labour. It is also released by the woman's body during orgasm and breastfeeding.

palpation The medical term for 'feeling' the baby within the uterus.

pelvimetry Estimating the size and shape of the pelvis using X-rays and palpation.

perinatal mortality rate (PMR or PNMR) The rate (usually expressed per 1,000) of babies dying between twenty-four weeks of pregnancy and seven days after birth.

perineal massage Massaging and stretching the perineum during pregnancy so as to reduce the risk of tearing or episiotomy during labour.

perineum The area of muscle between the vagina and anus.

physiotherapist A qualified health professional who treats people by physical means, including massage, manipulation, ultrasound and heat treatment. Obstetric physiotherapists have additional qualifications for working with women having babies.

placenta The organ which grows during pregnancy to supply the baby with food and oxygen from the mother's blood and to dispose of carbon dioxide via the umbilical cord.

placental abruption An emergency condition in which the placenta separates from the wall of the uterus either before or during labour before the baby has been born. Usually necessitates an emergency caesarean if severe.

placenta praevia A placenta sited in the lower part of the uterus. If over the cervix, the woman must be delivered by caesarean. In lesser degrees she may deliver vaginally in hospital.

postpartum haemorrhage The loss of more than 500 ml of blood by a woman after birth.

pre-eclampsia A condition arising during pregnancy which, if left untreated, could cause fits in the mother and cut off the oxygen supply to her baby. Symptoms are increased blood pressure often accompanied by swelling of the limbs and protein in the urine. The only 'cure' is delivery of the baby, often by caesarean if the condition is severe and the cervix unfavourable.

primigravida (sometimes shortened to 'primip') A woman having her first baby.

prognosis A medical estimate of the progress of a disease. Used to predict the ability of a woman to give birth vaginally.

protocol In a maternity unit, a written document specifying systems of care, such as the management of labour.

pulmonary embolism Part of a blood clot which detaches itself from a vein in the pelvis or leg and travels in the bloodstream to the lungs. A large embolus (clot which has detached itself) can cause immediate death.

registrar/senior registrar (doctors) A registrar is a qualified hospital doctor specialising in one area of medicine who hopes eventually to become a consultant. Senior registrars are usually very skilled and more experienced than registrars, ready to be consultants.

respiratory distress syndrome A condition occurring mainly in premature babies and in mature babies of diabetic mothers and those born by caesarean section. Babies with this condition have difficulty breathing and have to be connected to a machine to help them breathe.

senior house officer (SHO) Qualified doctors undergoing the practical part of their training. Some will go on to be hospital doctors, others GPs after the year spent as an SHO.

Sonicaid A portable instrument for checking the baby's heart rate during pregnancy and labour which works by ultrasound. Easy to use, whatever the position of the mother.

special care baby unit (SCBU) Hospital department where intensive care is given to babies by specially trained doctors and nurses using sophisticated equipment and techniques. Not every hospital has one and not every SCBU is able to look after babies who are so seriously ill as to need long-term ventilation in a neonatal intensive care unit.

spinal anaesthesia A form of local (regional) anaesthesia whereby an injection is given into the cerebrospinal fluid to numb the abdomen for a caesarean.

stages of labour First: from the beginning of labour until the cervix is 10 cm dilated. Second: the time from full dilatation to the birth of the baby. Third: the time during which the placenta is delivered.

sutures The medical word for stitches to repair a wound.

syntocinon Synthetic form of oxytocin used to make the uterus contract more strongly during induction or when spontaneous labour is thought to be progressing too slowly. Another trade name is pitocin.

syntometrine A mixture of the two drugs

syntocinon and ergometrine, used routinely in most hospitals to speed up delivery of the placenta and to reduce the risk of postpartum haemorrhage.

TENS (Transcutaneous Electrical Nerve Stimulation) A low-tech form of pain relief which a woman can use on herself by means of a small, hand-held, battery-operated machine. TENS work by means of two pairs of electrodes taped to the woman's lower back, transmitting a signal which works in two ways to reduce the level of pain from contractions. The first is by interfering with the signals being transmitted to the brain; the second by promoting the production of the body's naturally occurring pain-killers, endorphins.

transverse lie When the baby lies across the woman's body, rather than head- or bottom-down. Sometimes associated with a shoulder or arm presentation if not recognised until labour is advanced.

trial of labour Allowing a first-time mother to try to give birth vaginally when it is suspected that there may be feto-pelvic disproportion.

trial of scar Allowing a woman to try to give birth vaginally after a previous caesarean.

ultrasound scan Sound emitted at a frequency higher than the human ear can hear which bounces off the different parts of the mother's and baby's bodies at different rates, enabling an image of the baby inside the mother's body to appear on a screen.

umbilical cord This connects the baby to the placenta and is about 50 cm long. Two umbilical arteries carry blood from the mother to the baby and one umbilical vein carries blood from the baby to the mother.

variability The way in which the fetal heart rate responds to contractions and other stimuli.

VBAC Vaginal birth after caesarean.

Ventouse A method of helping a mother to deliver her baby, used by doctors. A cup is attached by a strong tube to an electric pump. The cup is put on the baby's head and a vacuum created by the pump to keep it in place. With one hand on the baby's head, the doctor pulls on the tube during a contraction to deliver the baby. If not much pulling is needed, a soft silicone cup can be used which causes less bruising to the baby's head. The mother may need a small episiotomy or none at all, depending on the position of the baby.

vitamin K A vitamin used by the liver to make the proteins needed to prevent haemorrhage. Routinely offered to most babies in the United Kingdom after birth to reduce the risks of haemorrhagic disease, a rare but often fatal disorder of the blood-clotting system.

BIBLIOGRAPHY

ACHCEW (1992), *A Health Standards Inspectorate*, Association of Community Health Councils for England and Wales and the Association for the Victims of Medical Accidents: London

AIMS (1991), 'VBAC: The right to a normal birth', *AIMS Journal*, vol. 4, no. 3

American College of Obstetricians and Gynecologists (1988), *Guidelines for Vaginal Delivery after a Previous Caesarean Birth*, Report by the Committee on Obstetrics: Washington DC

Anderson, G. M. and J. Lomas (1984), 'Determinants of the Increasing Cesarean Birth Rate', *New England Journal of Medicine*, vol. 311, pp. 887–92

Arney, W. A. (1982), in *Power and the Profession of Obstetrics*, University of Chicago Press: Chicago and London

Balaskas, J. (1989), *The New Active Birth*, Cambridge University Press: Cambridge

Balen, A. H. and J. M. Smith (1992), 'The CTG in Practice', Livingstone

Baliva, R. and A. Serpierri (1886), 'Extraordinary Caesarean Section', *The Lancet*, vol. 1, pp. 994–5.

Barrett, J. F. R., G. J. Jarvis, H. N. MacDonald, P. C. Buchan, S. N. Tyrrell and R. J. Lilford (1990). 'Inconsistencies in Clinical Decisions in Obstetrics', *The Lancet*, vol. 330, pp. 549–51

Baudelocque, M. (1801), *Two Memoirs on the Cesarean Operation*, trans. John Hull, Sowler and Russell: Manchester

Bell, G. (1916), 'Caesarean Section in a Pitman's Cottage', *British Medical Journal*, vol 1, pp. 195–6

Beukins, P., A. Tsui, M. Kotelchuck and J. Degraft-Johnson (1991), 'An Indicator of the Content of Prenatal Care in Developing Countries', in *International Conference on Primary Care Obstetrics and Perinatal Health*, Netherlands Institute of Primary Health Care: Utrecht

Blumenthal, N. J., R. S. Harris, M. C. O'Connor and P. A. L. Lancaster (1984), 'Changing Caesarean Section Rates: Experience at a Sydney obstetric teaching hospital', *The Australian and New Zealand Journal of Obstetrics and Gynaecology*, vol. 24, pp. 246–51

Boyd, C. and C. Francome (1983), *One Birth in Nine*, Maternity Alliance: London

Boylan, P. C. (1989), 'Active Management of Labor: Results in Dublin, Houston, London, New Brunswick, Singapore, and Valparaiso', *Birth*, vol. 16, no. 3, pp. 114–18

Bright Banister, J. (1935), 'Caesarean Section', *British Medical Journal*, vol. 2, pp. 684–5

British Medical Journal (1922), 'Caesarean Section', unsigned editorial, vol. 1, pp. 277–8.

British Medical Journal (1936), 'Caesarean Section', unsigned editorial, vol. 2, p. 1279–80

Butler, N. R. and D. G. Bonham (1963), *Perinatal Mortality*, Livingstone: Edinburgh and London

Canadian Conference (1986), *Final Statement of the Panel from the National Consensus Conference on Aspects of Cesarean Birth*, Planning Committee of the National Consensus Conference: Ontario

Carson, D. and C. Francome (1983), *Can We Avoid A Caesarean Crisis?*, Middlesex University: London

Chalmers, I., M. Enkin and M. J. N. C. Keirse (eds) (1989), *Effective Care in Pregnancy and Childbirth*, Oxford University Press: Oxford

Chamberlain, G. (1975), 'The First Week of Life', in Chamberlain and Chamberlain (eds)

Chamberlain, G. and A. Peattie (1991), *Annual Report of the Department of Obstetrics and Gynaecology*, St George's Hospital: London

Chamberlain, R. and G. Chamberlain (eds) (1975), *British Births*, Heinemann Medical Books: London

Clippingdale, S. D. (1911), 'The Accouchement of Queen Jane Seymour', *Journal of Obstetrics and Gynaecology of the British Empire*, pp. 109–16

Cohen, M. and B. S. Carson (1985), 'Respiratory Morbidity Benefit of Awaiting Onset of Labor after Elective Cesarean Section', *Obstetrics and Gynecology*, vol. 65, pp. 818–24

Collea, J. V., C. Chein and E. J. Quilligan (1980), 'The Randomised Management of Term Breech Presentation: A study of 208 cases', *American Journal of Obstetrics and Gynecology*, vol. 137, pp. 235–44

Coltart, T. M., J. A. Davies and M. Katesmark (1990), 'Outcome of a Second Pregnancy after a Previous Elective Caesarean Section', *British Journal of Obstetrics and Gynaecology*, vol. 97, pp. 1140–3

Cotgrove, S. A. and J. F. Norton (1942), 'Cesarean Section', *Journal of the American Medical Association*, vol. 118, no. 3, pp. 201–4

Craigin, E. (1916), 'Conservatism in Obstetrics', *New York State Journal of Medicine*, vol. 104, pp. 1–3

Davis, J. A. (1990), 'Doctors and Medical Negligence', *British Medical Journal*, vol. 300, pp. 746–7

Delee, J. B. (1913), *Principles and Practice of Obstetrics*, W. B. Saunders: Philadelphia and London

Delee, J. B. (1942), 'Cesarean Section', *Journal of the American Medical Association*, vol. 118, no. 3, pp. 201–9

DeMott, R. K. and H. F. Sandmire (1990), 'The Green Bay Cesarean Section Study', *American Journal of Obstetrics and Gynecology*, vol. 162, pp. 1593–602

Department of Health (1991), *Confidential Enquiries into Maternal Deaths in the United Kingdom 1985–87*, HMSO: London

DeRegt, R. H., H. L. Minkoff, J. Feldman and R. H. Schwarz (1986), 'Relation of Private or Clinic Care to the Cesarean Birth Rate', *New England Journal of Medicine*, vol. 315, pp. 619–24

Donald, I. (1955), *Practical Obstetric Problems*, Lloyd Luke: London

Durrand, A. M. (1992), 'The Safety of Home Birth: The Farm study', *Journal of the American Public Health Association*, vol. 82, pp. 450–2

Eden, T. W. and E. Holland (1931), *Manual of Midwifery*, 7th edn., Churchill: London

Eisenberg, H. (1986), 'A Doctor on Trial', *New York Times*, magazine section, 20 July, pp. 26–42

Enkin, M. W. (1991), 'Primary Care Obstetrics and Perinatal Health: Canada', International Conference on Primary Care Obstetrics and Perinatal Health, Netherlands Institute of Primary Health Care: Utrecht

Ferguson, I. L. C. (1985), 'Malpresentations and Malpositions', in J. W. Crawford (ed.), *Risks of Labour*, vol. 2, Wiley: Chichester

Ferriman, A. (1988), 'Op a Good Thing', *The Observer*, 31 July, p. 36.

Finney, Rev. P. A. (1935), *Moral Problems in Hospital Practice*, 5th edn., B. Herder Book Company: London

Flamm, B. L. (1985), 'Vaginal Birth after Cesarean Section: Controversies old and new', *Clinics in Obstetrics and Gynecology*, vol. 28, pp. 735–44

Flamm, B. (1992), 'Should Electronic Fetal Monitoring Always be Used for Women in Labor who are Having a Vaginal Birth after a Previous Caesarean?' *Birth*, vol. 19, no. 1, pp. 31–2

Francome, C. (1984), *Abortion Freedom*, Unwin Hyman: London and Boston

Francome, C. (1990a), *Sane New World*, Carla Publications: London

Francome, C. (1990b), *Changing Childbirth*, Maternity Alliance: London

Francome, C. and P. J. Huntingford, 'Births by Caesarean Section in the United States of America and Britain', *Journal of Biosocial Science*, vol. 12, pp. 353–62

Frigoletto, F. D., K. J. Ryan and M. Phillippe (1980), 'Maternal Mortality Rate Associated with Cesarean Section: An appraisal', *American Journal of Obstetrics and Gynecology*, vol. 136, pp. 969–70

Giesen, D. (1993), 'Legal Accountability for the Provision of Health Care: A comparative view', unpublished paper presented at the

Royal Society of Medicine Forum on Quality in Health Care, 10 February

Gleicher, N. (1984), 'Cesarean Section Rates in the United States', *Journal of the American Medical Association*, vol. 252, pp. 3273–6

Gould, J. B., M. P. H. Becky Davey and R. S. Stafford (1989), 'Socioeconomic Differences in Rates of Cesarean Section', *New England Journal of Medicine*, vol. 321, pp. 233–9

Goyert, G. L., S. F. Bottoms, M. C. Treadwell and P. C. Nehra (1989), 'The Physician Factor in Cesarean Birth Rates', *New England Journal of Medicine*, vol. 320, pp. 706–9

Green, J. M., V. A. Coupland and J. V. Kitzinger (1988), *Great Expectations: A Prospective Study of Women's Expectations and Experiences of Childbirth*, unpublished report for the Health Promotion Research Trust and the Nuffield Provincial Hospital Trust

Griffin, J. (1993), *Born Too Soon*, Office of Health Economics: London

Guillimeau, J. (1612), *Childbirth*, A. Hatfield: London

Hamilton, Alexander (1803), *Outlines of the Theory and Practice of Midwifery*, 5th edn., T. Kay: Edinburgh

Hansell, R. S., K. B. McMurray and G. R. Huey (1990), 'Vaginal Birth after Two or More Cesarean Sections: A five year experience', *Birth*, vol. 17, no. 3, pp. 146–50

Harris, R. P. (1880), *American Journal of Medical Science*, vol. 78, p. 43

Harris, R. P. (1980a), 'The Porro Modification of the Cesarean Operation in Continental Europe', *American Journal of Medical Science*, vol. 79, pp. 335–62

Harris, R. P. (1980b), 'The Results of the First 50 Cases of Cesarean Ovaro-hysterectomy 1869–80', *American Journal of Medical Science*, vol. 80, pp. 129–34

Hausknecht, R. and J. R. Heilman (1978), *Having A Cesarean Baby*, Dutton: New York

Health Committee (1992), *Maternity Services*, House of Commons, Second Report, HMSO: London

Hemminki, E., B. I. Graubard, H. J. Hoffmann, W. D. Mosher and K. Fetterly (1985), 'Cesarean and Subsequent Fertility: Results from the 1982 National Survey of Family Growth', *American Fertility Society*, vol. 43, no. 4, pp. 520–8

Hillan, E. M. (1992a), 'Maternal–Infant Attachment Following Caesarean Delivery', *Journal of Clinical Nursing*, vol. 1, no. 1, pp. 33–7

Hillan, E. M. (1992b), 'Short Term Morbidity Associated with Cesarean Delivery', *Birth*, vol. 19, pp. 190–4

Hofmeyr, G. J. (1991), 'External Cephalic Version at Term: How high are the stakes?', *British Journal of Obstetrics and Gynaecology*, vol. 98, pp. 1–3

Hofmeyr, G. J. and M. J. N. C. Keirse (1990), 'Two Ways to Reduce Caesarean Section Rates', Oxford Database of Perinatal Trials, *Newsletter*, 1–4 August

Holland, E. (1920), 'Rupture of Caesarean Section Scar', *British Medical Journal*, vol. 1, pp. 705–7

Hull, John (1798), *A Defence of the Caesarean Operation*, R. & W. Dean: Manchester

Inch, S. (1989), *Birthrights*, Greenprint: London

Janowich, B., M. S. Nakamwa, L. F. Entellita, M. L. Brown and D. Clapton (1982), 'Caesarian Section in Brazil', *Social Science and Medicine*, vol. 16, pp. 19–25

Johnstone, R. W. (1952), *Midwifery*, 15th edn., Adam and Charles Black: London

Kaufman, K. (1990), 'Commentary: Midwifery in Ontario', *Birth*, vol. 17, no. 3, p. 144

Kennell, J., M. Klaus, S. McGrath, S. S. Robertson and C. Hinckley (1991), 'Continuous Emotional Support during Labor in a US Hospital', *Journal of the American Medical Association*, vol. 17, pp. 2197–201

Kerr, J. M. M. (1937), *Operative Obstetrics*, 4th edn., Baillière Tindall and Cox: London

Kerr, J. M. M., J. H. Ferguson, J. Young and J. Hendry (1933), *A Combined Textbook of Obstetrics and Gynaecology*, 2nd edn., Livingstone: Edinburgh

Krishnamurthy, S., F. Fairlie, A. D. Cameron, J. J. Walker and J. R. MacKenzie (1991), 'The Role of Postnatal X-ray Pelvimetry after

Caesarean Section in the Management of Subsequent Delivery', *British Journal of Obstetrics and Gynaecology*, vol. 98, pp. 716–18

Lao, T. T., B. F. H. Leung and S. S. Young (1987), 'Trial of Scar: Is it safe in developing countries?', *British Journal of Clinical Practice*, vol. 41, no. 2, pp. 596–600

Lavin, J., R. Stephens, M. Miodovnik and T. Barden (1982), 'Vaginal Delivery in Patients with a Prior Caesarean Section', *Obstetrics and Gynecology*, vol. 59, p. 135

Levene, M. I. (1986), 'Grand Multiple Pregnancies and Demand for Neonatal Intensive Care', *The Lancet*, vol. 2, pp. 347–8

Lewison, H. (1991), *Your Choices for Pregnancy and Childbirth*, Ebury Press: London

Lilford, R. J., H. A. Van Coeverden De Groot and P. J. Moore (1990), 'The Relative Risks of Caesarean Section and Vaginal Delivery', *British Journal of Obstetrics and Gynaecology*, vol. 97, pp. 882–92

Lomas, J. (1988), 'Holding Back the Tide of Caesareans', *British Medical Journal*, vol. 297, pp. 569–70

Lomas, J. (1991), 'Words Without Actions? The production, dissemination and impact of consensus recommendations', *Annual Review of Public Health*, vol. 12, pp. 41–65

Lomas, J. and M. Enkin (1989), 'Variations in Operative Delivery Rates', in Chalmers, Enkin and Keirse, pp. 1182–95

Mabie, W. C., J. R. Barton and N. Wasserstrumn (1992), 'Clinical Observations on Asthma in Pregnancy', *Journal of Maternal and Fetal Medicine*, vol. 1, no. 1, pp. 45–50

MacDonald, D. (1992), 'Should Electronic Fetal Monitoring Always be Used for Women in Labor who are Having a Vaginal Birth after a Previous Caesarean?', *Birth*, vol. 19, no. 1, p. 31–2

MacDonald, D., A. Grant, M. Sheridan-Pereira, P. Boylan and I. Chalmers (1985), 'The Dublin random controlled trial of intrapartum fetal heart rate monitoring', *American Journal of Obstetrics and Gynecology*, vol. 152, pp. 524–39

Maternity Services (1992), *Government Response to the Second Report from the Health Select Committee*, Cmmd. 2018, HMSO: London

McIlroy, Dame Louise (1932), 'Indications For and Against Caesarean Section', *British Medical Journal*, vol. 2, pp. 796–7

McIlwaine, G. M., S. K. Cole and M. C. Macnaughton (1985), 'The Rising Caesarean Section Rate: A matter of concern', *Health Bulletin*, vol. 43, pp. 301–4

McIntosh-Marshall, C. (1949), 'Modern Caesarean Section', *British Medical Journal*, vol. 2, p. 147

Molloy, B. G., O. Sheil and N. M. Duignan (1987), 'Delivery after Caesarean Section: Review of 2,176 consecutive cases', *British Medical Journal*, vol. 294, pp. 1645–6

Murray-Arthur, F. and J. F. Correy (1984), 'A Review of Primary Caesarean Sections in Tasmania', *The Australian and New Zealand Journal of Obstetrics and Gynaecology*, vol. 24, p. 242

National Childbirth Trust (1992), *Maternity Services Survey*, London

National Consensus Conference on Aspects of Cesarean Birth (1986), *Final Statement of Panel*, presented by Planning Committee and Dr W. Hannah, Panel Chairman

National Institutes of Health (1982), *Cesarean Childbirth*, US Department of Health and Human Services, Public Health Service, Publication No. 82–2067, US Government Printing Office: Washington DC

Newburn, M. (1993), 'NCT 1992 Maternity Services Survey', *New Generation*, vol. 12, no. 2

Newell, F. S. (1921), *Cesarean Section*, D. Appleton: New York and London

NHS Management Executive (1993), *A Study of Midwife and GP Led Maternity Units*, London

Oakley, A. and M. Richards (1990), 'Women's Experiences of Caesarean Delivery', in *The Politics of Maternity Care*, ed. J. Garcia, R. Kilpatrick and M. Richards, Oxford University Press: Oxford

O'Driscoll, K. and M. Foley (1983), 'Correlation of Decrease in Perinatal Mortality and Increase in Cesarean Section Rates', *Journal of the American College of Obstetrics and Gynecology*, vol. 61, no. 1, pp. 1–5

Office of Population Censuses and Surveys (1990), *Mortality Statistics – Perinatal and Infant: Social and Biological Factors in England and Wales*, HMSO: London.

Office of Population Censuses and Surveys (1992), *1990 'Infant Feeding'*, HMSO: London

Olofsson, P. and H. Rhydstrom (1985), 'Twin Delivery: How should the second twin be delivered?', *American Journal of Obstetrics and Gynecology*, vol. 153, pp. 479–81

Omu, A. E. (1991), 'Reducing Perinatal Mortality in Nigeria through Primary Obstetric Care', International Conference on Primary Care Obstetrics and Perinatal Health, Netherlands Institute of Primary Care: Utrecht, p. 70

Perez, P. G. (1989), 'The Patient Observer: What really led to these cesarean births?', *Birth*, vol. 16, no. 3, pp. 130–9

Phaff, J. M. L. (1986), 'The Organisation and Administration of Perinatal Services in the Netherlands', in *Perinatal Health Services in Europe*, Croom Helm: London and Sydney, pp. 117–27

Phelan, J. P., M. O. Ahn and F. Diaz (1989), 'Twice a Caesarean Always a Caesarean', *Obstetrics and Gynecology*, vol. 73, pp. 161–5

Philipp, E. (1988), *Caesareans*, Sidgwick & Jackson: London

Placek, P. J., S. M. Taffel and M. Moien (1988), '1986 C-sections Rise: VBACs inch upward', *American Journal of Public Health*, vol. 78, no. 5, pp. 562–3

Playfair, W. S. (1886), *The Science and Practice of Midwifery*, 6th edn., Smith, Elder: London

Porreco, R. P. (1990), 'The Twice Wounded Uterus', *Birth*, vol. 17, no. 3, pp. 150–1

Quinn, M. (1993), 'Fax Transmission from the Labour Ward', *Hospital Update Plus*, April, pp. 64–6.

Radford, Thomas (1865), *Observations on the Caesarean Section and on Other Obstetric Operations*, T. Richards: London

Read, A. W., W. J. Waddell, W. J. Prendiville and F. J. Stanley (1991), *Caesarean Section and Operative Vaginal Delivery in Western Australia 1981–7*, International Conference on Primary Care Obstetrics and Perinatal Health, Netherlands Institute of Primary Care: Utrecht, p. 45

Redman, C. and I. Walker (1992), *Pre-eclampsia: The facts – the hidden threat to pregnancy*, Oxford University Press: Oxford

Renwick, M. Y. (1991), *The Australian and New Zealand Journal of Obstetrics and Gynaecology*, vol. 31, no. 4, pp. 299–304

Rooks, J. P., N. L. Weatherby, E. K. M. Ernst, S. Stapleton, D. Rosen and A. Rosenfield (1989), 'Outcomes of Care in Birth Centres', *New England Journal of Medicine*, vol. 321, pp. 1804–11

Routh, A. (1911), 'On Caesarean Section in the United Kingdom', *Journal of Obstetrics and Gynaecology of the British Empire*, vol. 19, pp. 1–25

Royal College of Midwives (1991), *Successful Breastfeeding*, 2nd edn., Livingstone: London

Rydhstrom, H., I. Ingemarsson and S. Ohrlander (1990), 'Lack of Correlation Between a High Caesarean Section Rate and Improved Prognosis for Low-Birthweight Twins (2500g)', *British Journal of Obstetrics and Gynaecology*, vol. 97, pp.229–36

Sanchez-Ramos, L., A. M. Kaunitz, H. B. Peterson, B. Martinez-Schnell and R. J. Thompson (1990), 'Reducing Cesarean Sections at a Teaching Hospital', *American Journal of Obstetrics and Gynecology*, vol. 163, pp. 1081–8

Savage, W. (1986), *A Savage Enquiry: Who Controls Childbirth?*, Virago: London.

Savage, W. (1990), 'Technology-free Obstetrics at Semmelweis Clinic', *The Lancet*, vol. 336, p. 178

Savage, W. and C. Francome (1993), 'British Caesarean Rates: Have we reached a plateau?', *British Journal of Obstetrics and Gynaecology*, vol. 100, pp. 493–6

Schroeder, C. (1873), *Manual of Midwifery*, 3rd edn., trans. C. H. Carter, Churchill: London

Shearer, E. (1992), 'Should Electronic Fetal Monitoring Always be Used for Women in Labor who are Having a Vaginal Birth after a Previous Caesarean?', *Birth*, vol. 19, no. 1, pp. 33–4

Shulte, A. J. (1917), quoted in the *Critic and Guide*, New York, p. 52

Simkin, P. (1991), 'Just Another Day in a Woman's Life: Women's long-term perception of their first birth experience', *Birth*, vol. 18, no. 4, pp. 203–10

Simmons, W. (1799), 'Reflection on the Propriety of Performing the Caesarean Operation', *The Medical and Physical Journal*, vol. 2, p. 231

Smith, R. (1990), 'The Epidemiology of Malpractice', *British Medical Journal*, vol. 301, pp. 621–2

Spastics Society (1992), *Paying for Disability: No-fault Compensation – Panacea or Pandora's Box?*, London

Stembera, Z. (1987), 'Epidemiology of Perinatal Statistics', *Cesk-Gynekol*, vol. 52, no. 2, pp. 162–4

Stembera, Z. (1992), 'Development of Indications for Cesarean Section in the Czech Republic', *Cas-lek-Cesk*, vol. 131, no. 8, pp. 225–30

Stephenson, P. A. (1992), *International Difference in the Use of Obstetric Interventions*, World Health Organization: Copenhagen

Stewart, D. (1747), 'The Caesarean Operation Done with Success by a Midwife', *Medical Essays and Observations*, 3rd edn., pt. 1, pp. 360–2

Sutherst, J. R. and B. D. Case (1975), 'Caesarean Section and Its Place in the Active Approach to Delivery', *Clinics in Obstetrics and Gynaecology*, vol. 2, no. 1, pp. 241–61

Taffel, S. M., P. J. Placek and C. L. Kosary (1992), 'US Cesarean Section Rates 1990: An update', *Birth*, vol. 19, no. 1, pp. 21–2

Theobold, G. W. (1949), 'Modern Caesarean Section', *British Medical Journal*, vol. 2, p. 147

Treffers, P. E. and R. Laan (1986), 'Regional Perinatal Mortality and Regional Hospitalisation of Delivery in the Netherlands', *British Journal of Obstetrics and Gynaecology*, vol. 93, pp. 690–3

Tweedy, H. (1911), 'Caesarean Section and Its Alternatives', *British Medical Journal*, vol. 1, pp. 496–8

Van Teijlingen, E. R. (1990), 'The Profession of Maternity Home Care Assistant and its Significance for the Dutch Midwifery Profession', *International Journal of Nursing Studies*, vol. 27, no. 4, pp. 355–66

Whitridge, W. J. (1921), 'A Critical Analysis of 212 Years Experience with Caesarean Section', *Johns Hopkins Hospital Bulletin*, vol. 32, p. 173

Woodcock, H., A. W. Read, D. J. Moore, F. J. Stanley and C. Bower (1991), 'An Epidemiological Comparison of Planned Home and Hospital Births in Western Australia 1981–1987', International Conference on Primary Care Obstetrics and Perinatal Health, Netherlands Institute of Primary Health Care

World Health Organization (1985), 'Appropriate Technology for Birth', *The Lancet*, vol. 331, pp. 436–7

Wright, E. A., M. M. Kapu and H. I. Onwuhafua (1991), 'Perinatal Mortality and Cesarean Section in Jos University Teaching Hospital', *International Journal of Gynaecology and Obstetrics*, vol. 35, no. 4, pp. 299–304

Young, G. (1987), 'Are Isolated Maternity Units run by General Practitioners Dangerous?', *British Medical Journal*, vol. 294, pp. 744–7

Young, J. H. (1944), *Caesarean Section: The History and Development of the Operation from the Earliest Times*, H. K. Lewis: London

Zuspan, F. P., E. J. Quilligan, J. D. Iams and H. P. van Geijn (1979), 'Predictors in Intrapartum Fetal Distress: The role of electronic fetal monitoring', *American Journal of Obstetrics and Gynecology*, vol. 135, pp. 287–91

FURTHER INFORMATION FOR PARENTS

Reading

Balaskas, J., *The New Active Birth*, Unwin, 1989
How to prepare for an active birth.

Enkin, M., M. Keirse and I. Chalmers, *A Guide to Effective Care in Pregnancy and Childbirth*, Oxford University Press, 1990
A summary of research findings on all aspects of maternity care.

Inch, S., *Birthrights*, Greenprint, 1989
A critical review of hospital procedures which in many units have become routine.

Smale, M., *The NCT Book of Breastfeeding*, Vermillion, 1992
A straightforward, reassuring guide to breastfeeding.

Tucker, G., *The NCT Book of Pregnancy, Birth and Parenthood*, Oxford University Press, 1992
A comprehensive manual for parents on preparing for birth and what to expect.

A number of specialised leaflets on breastfeeding, including breastfeeding after a caesarean, are available from NCT (Maternity Sales) Limited (see below for the address).

Organisations

Association for Improvements in the Maternity Services (AIMS), 40 Kingswood Avenue, London NW6 6LS, Tel. 081-960 5585
Voluntary pressure group offering support with regard to parents' rights, complaints procedures and choices for maternity care.

Association for Post-natal Illness (APNI), 25 Jerdan Place, London SW6 1BE, Tel. 071-386 0868
Network of volunteers who have suffered from postnatal illness and offer information and support.

Caesarean Support Network, c/o Sheila Tunstall, 2 Hurst Park Drive, Huyton, Liverpool L36 1TF, Tel. 051-480 1184
Offers emotional support and practical advice to women who have had or may need a caesarean.

National Childbirth Trust, Alexandra House, Oldham Terrace, Acton, London W3 6NH, Tel. 081-992 8637.
Nearly 400 branches throughout the United Kingdom with networks of informal support, including antenatal teachers, breastfeeding counsellors and postnatal support groups. Local branches will have information about what sort of service to expect from local maternity services and will have details of local support groups for home birth and for women who have had or are expecting to have a caesarean. ParentAbility provides information for parents with disabilities or medical conditions and puts them in touch with each other.

NCT (Maternity Sales) Limited, Burnfield Avenue, Glasgow G46 7TL, Tel. 041-633 5552 (Fax 041-633 5677)
Supplies a wide range of books, leaflets and maternity goods, including nursing bras and the famous NCT stretch briefs, by mail order. Catalogue available.

Stillbirth and Neonatal Death Society (SANDS), 28 Portland Place, London W1N 4DE, Tel. 071-436 5881
Information and a national network of support groups for parents who have lost a baby.

VBAC Information and Support, c/o Linda Howes, 8 Wren Way, Farnborough, Hants, Tel. 0252-543250
Network of volunteers offering information and support for women wanting a vaginal birth after a previous caesarean.

INDEX